# IVF

# A DETAILED GUIDE

Everything I Wish I Had Known
Before Starting My Fertility
Treatments

BIANCA SMITH

D0681739

# DEDICATION

**The love of my life, my soul mate, my best friend, my hero, my everything, my husband, Vincent Smith. There are not enough words that exist to express my love and gratitude for you, the perfect person for me.**

# WHY I CREATED THIS BOOK

Twelve years ago at the age of 29, the fun of family planning was abruptly forced into an alternate reality filled with the coldness of embryo planning instead.

I thought (as ones does) that it would take a few months of intimate copulation between two people who loved each other to create beautiful little replicas of both husband and wife. Instead it became many more than a few years of clinical, meticulously timed, medicated probing sessions between wife; and a range of doctors, nurses, surgeons, embryologists, anesthetists, sometimes even students, and every now and then a husband to create little fertilised embryos – and that's just 1 aspect of 9,999 other challenging aspects when it comes to the business of assisted reproductive technology (ART) in any form.

When I was kicked in the head by the beast that is infertility, it left me upside down and inside out in a black world of confusion, ignorance, despair, isolation, pain and suffering. I faced an enemy that I had absolutely no idea how to fight and neither did anyone else I knew at that time.

# WHAT THIS BOOK IS ABOUT & WHY IT IS FOR YOU

This book is a handy guide for those trying to conceive, specifically through assisted reproduction treatment with a few extra tips and suggestions to make your journey a little richer.

It is primarily a collation of fundamental information that my husband and I would have wished for when we first started our IVF journey. If we had known even half the things we know today, we would have been so much better prepared for what was coming.

I personally spent years drudging through a swamp of overwhelming materials, had countless conversations with medical practitioners as well as couples who had been through what we were going through, made a number of hard-learnt mistakes and wasted heaps of money and tears to learn what I know now about ART, specifically invitro fertilisation (IVF).

A resource book would have been a lighthouse while I sailed through the dark and so I put together this guide, to equip other individuals or couples embarking on and also still in the middle of this journey with at least the basic knowledge they need to navigate the rough seas of fertility treatments and IVF.

The information in this book is only a fraction of all the information out there. Although there are medically factual segments, this is not a medical journal and everything must always be discussed with a certified medical practitioner first. All the suggestions are also just suggestions and don't claim to be the only road to Rome. The clinics and service providers featured are based on personal preference and or/experiences from other ladies on this journey that I have spoken to, and not on any documented statistics.

Also note that I have not received any sort of compensation from any service provider mentioned as part of paid advertising or any other promotion.

All information is merely an attempt to bring together everything that I have learnt along the way to make life a little easier for you on your journey than it was for me and I sincerely hope it will do exactly that for you.

I was living in the UK during all my IVF treatments; therefore this book will have the UK as a frame of reference, however, most of the information in this book is generic and the country shouldn't make much of a difference in general.

I hope that you will find this guide useful and I wish you all the luck in the world on your journey. It's not an easy journey, but I guarantee that with this guide, much of your initial stress in knowing where to start and what route to pursue will be eliminated.

Please feel free to contact me via email to *mrsbinkysmith@gmail.com* at any time should you have questions or just need to chat with someone who has been there.

I would like to thank everyone who was involved in any way in my life in a positive manner – my husband, my friends, the many ladies in all my on-line support groups and my family, as well as everyone who was involved in the creation of this book and specifically:

❖ My fabulous, amazing, wonderful and gorgeous life coach and friend, Rosanne Austin of From Maybe to Baby (**http://www.frommaybetobaby.com**), who has patiently worked with me to bring out my talents and my strengths and helped to get to a point of loving my life no matter what! Without her, I wouldn't have put this book together!

❖ My beautiful, talented, gracious friend, Rachel Campbell of Sprout & Co (**http://www.sproutandco.com.au**) who has been a major contributor to my journey and this Book in so many ways, and whose friendship is so precious to me.

❖ My amazing, sweet, incredible friend, Monica Bivas of The IVF Journey (**http://monicabivas.com**), who is an absolute angel, inspiration and source of encouragement to myself and all who meet her.

❖ The fantastic, lovely, huge-hearted Kate Davies of Your Fertility Journey (**http://yourfertilityjourney.com**), who always goes above and beyond to give everyone she meets on this journey a personal touch of love, support and as much of her expert knowledge as she can.

❖ The very funny, wise, nurturing and deliciously crazy Lori Shandle-Fox, author of Laughing IS Conceivable (**http://laughingisconceivable.com**), who I was so blessed to have interviewed for my blog and even more blessed to now have as a friend.

❖ **All the absolutely awesome, magnificent, brave, inspirational, encouraging, fearless, loving and caring warrior women from all my online support groups**, without which I wouldn't have been able to get through my dark days in one piece. I am so thrilled to have met these wonderful souls on my journey and proud to call many of them close friends. There are too many to mention here and I would hate to forget a name by mistake, so you better know who you are because I love you and thank you all.


*With love,*
*Bianca*

# COMMONLY USED IVF ABBREVIATIONS

The following words with their abbreviations will be useful when visiting personal blogs or joining any sort of online support group. They are not medical terms but are frequently used amongst women/ couples trying to conceive. Don't worry if they seem overwhelming at first, you will use these enough times on your journey and be abbreviating like a pro!

**2ww** – 2 week wait – the time between embryo transfer and pregnancy test

**AF** – Aunt Flo – that time of the month

**AH** – Assisted Hatching

**AI** – Artificial Insemination

**AMH** – Anti-Mullerian Hormone (level of ovarian reserve)

**ART** – Assisted Reproductive Technology

**BA** – Baby Aspirin

**BBs** – Boobs / Breasts

**BBT** – Basal Body Temperature

**BCP** – Birth Control Pills

**BD** – Baby Dance (intercourse)

**Beta** – Blood Pregnancy Test checking your HCG levels

**BFN** – Big Fat Negative (pregnancy test)

**BFP** – Big Fat Positive (pregnancy test)

**B/W** – Blood Work

**CD** – Cycle Day

**CM** – Cervical Mucus

**D&C** – Dilation & Curettage

**DE** – Donor Eggs

**DH** – Dear Husband

**DOR** – Diminished Ovarian Reserve

Everything I wish I had Known Before Starting My Fertility Treatments

**DPO** – Days Past Ovulation

**DPT** – Days Past Transfer

**1DP3DT** – 1 Day Past a 3-Day Transfer

**ENDO** – Endometriosis

**ER** – Egg Retrieval

**ERPC** – Evacuation of Retained Products of Conception

**ET** – Embryo Transfer

**E2** - Estradiol

**FET** – Frozen Embryo Transfer

**FMU** – First Morning Urine

**FRER** – First Response Early Result (home pregnancy test)

**Frostie** – Frozen Embryo

**FSH** – Follicle Stimulating Hormone

**FXed** – Fingers Crossed

**GP** – General Practitioner (family doctor)

**HCG** – Human Chorionic Gonadotropin

**HPT** – Home Pregnancy Test

**HRT** – Hormone Replacement Therapy

**HSC** – Hysteroscopy

**HSG** – Hysterosalpinogram

**IB** – Implantation Bleeding

**ICSI** – Intra-Cytoplasmic Sperm Injection

**IF** – Infertility

**IM** – Intramuscular Injection

**Intralipids** – Intravenous Drip to combat auto-immune problems

**IUI** – Intra-Uterine Insemination

**IVF** – In Vitro Fertilization

**IVIg** – Intravenous Immunoglobulin

**LAP** – Laparoscopy

**LMP** – Last Menstrual Period (start date)

**LSC** – Low Sperm Count

**M/C** – Miscarriage

**MF** – Male Factor

**MIL** – Mother-In-Law

**MMC** – Missed Miscarriage

**NK Cells** – Natural Killer Cells

**OB/GYN** – Obstetrician/Gynecologist

**OH** – Other Half

**OHSS** – Ovarian Hyperstimulation Syndrome

**OPK** – Ovulation Prediction Kit

**OV** – Ovulation

**PCOS** – Polycystic Ovary Syndrome

**PGD/PGS** – Pre-implantation Genetic Diagnosis/Pre-Implantation Genetic Screening (testing an embryo pre-transfer for genetic diseases, such as Down's syndrome or cystic fibrosis)

**POAS** – Peeing On A Stick (home pregnancy test)

**RE** – Reproductive Endocrinologist (fertility doctor)

**SA** – Semen Analysis

**SIL** – Sister-in-law

**Snowbabies** – Frozen Embryos (also called frosties)

**Stimming** – Starting injectable medications for IVF cycle

**TIA** – Thanks in Advance

**TMI** – Too Much Information

**TTC** – Trying To Conceive

# CONTENTS

# 1 CHECKLIST FOR CONCEIVING THE NATURAL (TRADITIONAL) WAY

After six months of simply having regular unprotected sex, I suggest you first explore the natural way a bit more before you move onto expensive tests and even further for treatments.

Speaking from experience, I can tell you that the natural way often isn't all that natural when your main goal is to get pregnant.

The natural way means making sure that you have intercourse in the exact fertile window specific to your body, which doesn't necessarily stay the same each month. Generally women have around 4 days in their fertile window. During these 4 days, you need to have intercourse each day so that you don't accidentally miss your ovulation. Once you ovulate, the egg only lives for 12 to 24 hours in which time you should make sure that at least one of those swimmers is waiting in the fallopian tube to meet the egg when it falls.

Sound easy?

Yes, sure it does. All you're doing is having a lot of sex that you normally have any way, so you're having fun while trying to conceive.

Nope.

Having sex day after day because you have to, you have been told to and the only reason why you are having sex on these particular days is to procreate – is controlled fun and therefore not all that much fun. That is pressure, monotony and frustration.

However, before looking at any possible tests, medications and invasive treatments, here's a quick look at what you need and then I'll go into a few of them in a little more detail.

*1 Digital Basal Thermometer (with 2 decimal places):* these are very cheap and can be bought from many online retailers. Try to get one that lights up so you can see it in the dark. Also, a great idea would be to choose one that has a memory function. In this way you can quickly take your temperature at the same time even when you want to have an extra hour of sleep – when you wake you can check what your last reading was and record it.

*2 LH surge Test Kit or Ovulation Prediction Kit (OPK):* Available from most major retailers in store and online, from the very cheap to rather expensive.

*3 Saliva-based Fertility Test:* There are various options available online, all similarly priced. I use Fertile Focus which was £25 ($36 USD) from Amazon. It's pretty flimsy and I already cracked it within my first week but it carried on working with no problem.

*4 Sperm-friendly Lubricant:* There are a few names going around, but I personally wouldn't use anything other than Pre-Seed. Available online and at some pharmacies.

*5 A fully-integrated ovulation App:* Download from the app store to your smart phone. My personal favourite is Fertility Friend, who also sends you daily tutorials on everything you need to know for checking ovulation from cervical fluid or cervical mucus (CM) to oestrogen and progesterone in the body but do be aware of the predicted ovulation date (double check this through other methods) as they aren't always accurate with these.

*6 An online support group* that specialises in trying to conceive naturally with experts offering valuable advice, such as Your Fertility Support Group, which is run by Kate Davies, an experienced Fertility Nurse and Fertility Coach in the UK. Kate provides a wealth of information on things like ovulation. More details can be found in the chapter entitled Support Groups and under the Resources Page of this book.

Let's look at these in more detail...

**Basal Thermometer**

Why?

Your basal body temperature (BBT) is your temperature when your body is fully at rest. During ovulation, your temperature always increases slightly. Your most fertile days are usually the 2 or 3 days before your temperature rise. A temperature rise indicates that ovulation has already occurred. Temperature charting might also tell you whether you are pregnant before a positive pregnancy test. After ovulation, a rise in your basal temperature that lasts 18 days or longer could be an early sign.

How?

- Make sure your thermometer is always within easy reach next to your bed.
- Set your alarm for the same time each morning.
- Slip your thermometer under your tongue and wait for it to beep before getting out of bed or moving around.
- If you don't have a thermometer with a memory function, then make a note of your reading - include the date, time and day of your cycle. I usually make note of these on my phone which is also always next to me. You can print out one of the many free fertility charts on the internet, add your figures every day and draw your graph, or you can download one of the free apps onto your smart phone.
- At the same time as you are charting your temperature, you should be noting your cervical mucus and when you had intercourse. There will be fields to enter this information on both the printed charts and the app. Cervical mucus is without a doubt the most accurate ovulation indicator. Whenever a woman notices cervical mucus (fertile or not) she is always potentially fertile and this is because the sperm can live up to 5 (on some occasions 7) days in the vagina.

**Note on Cervical Mucus (CM)**

As your hormone levels change during your cycle, the amount, texture and colour of your mucus also changes. By keeping track of your cervical mucus, you can cross-reference the changes with your other fertility tracking methods to find out when your most fertile days are.

During your period:
menstrual blood

Just after your period:
dry for a few days and then becomes cloudy & sticky

Fertile Window:
clear, slippery or like egg-white in colour and consistency and it increases in volume (this is your body making it easier for sperm to travel through your cervix and to your egg)

High Fertile Days:
clear mucus strings which you can stretch between your fingers

Most Fertile Days:
very slippery & very watery

Fertile Window over:
dry, cloudy or sticky

Just before period:
a little watery or dry days again

**My Positive Points on using a Basal Thermometer:**

- It's cheap.
- It's exciting to learn how your body works once you start seeing a
- pattern and you can try to predict the next phase your body is moving into.

**My negative points on using a Basal Thermometer:**

- Your readings will be wrong if you don't get at least 4 hours sleep, or if you sleep in, if you're sick, if you've had medication including pain pills or have had alcohol. Although you can discount this if you make a note and learn what you need to look out for.
- Due to the above points, it's not always accurate and therefore needs to be used in conjunction with other fertility kits, but again, if you learn this method well you can overcome this.
- It will take a few months to work out your body's pattern.
- Sometimes our bodies rebel and refuse to follow usual patterns.
- Daily charting can become tedious.
- A lot of women use this method but don't actually know how to interpret the data. Therefore seeing a fertility specialist to help them is preferable.

## LH SURGE TEST KIT OR OVULATION PREDICTION KIT (OPK)

Why?

LH stands for Luteinizing Hormone. A rise of LH in women triggers ovulation.

In order for an egg to be fertilised, sperm needs to be waiting in the fallopian tubes for the egg or it needs to meet the egg head on as it moves down the tubes. Therefore it is important to know when you are going to ovulate before you actually ovulate. A good way to know this is to use an LH test kit.

These are all urine tests and they can range from plain paper strips to fancy digital contraptions with prices ranging from pocket change to pulling money from your savings.

The important thing to know is what works for you. As with every single step in TTC, every woman is different and what works perfectly for one might not work at all for another. Play around with a few different types and see what works best. You need to find what works for YOU.


How?


If you have regular cycles that run from 25 to 32 days, it is recommended that for your first month, you start testing on Day 10 of your cycle (with Day 1 being the first day of your full period flow).

You will most likely find that your LH surge will only be somewhere between Day 14 and Day 18 of your cycle, however, as everyone's body works differently, you won't know what day your surge is until you test it out. The most important lesson on this fertility journey is NEVER ASSUME ANYTHING.

Before peeing on your stick, read the instructions for your particular set of sticks. Some people will advise to test with your first morning urine (FMU) while others will say lunch time and others still will say later in the afternoon. So best to check what the instructions for YOUR tests say and follow those.

Once you get your LH Surge, you are at peak fertility and will generally ovulate between 12 and 48 hours thereafter, so it is essential to have intercourse as soon as you get the surge to make sure the sperm is ready for the egg and still the next few days after that just to make sure.

**My Positive Points on LH Surge Tests or OPK's:**

- There's a range – from very cheap to quite expensive
- If you ovulate, then the surge will be obvious. You will notice just before you surge as the lines on the (non-digital stick) won't be an exact match in shade – it is highly advisable to have intercourse at this time. You will notice when you are surging as the lines will be an exact match in shade – definitely have intercourse at this time.
- Because an LH surge happens before you actually ovulate, it is a good way to make sure that you don't miss your ovulation window if you are testing regularly.

**My negative points on LH Surge Tests or OPK's:**

- The LH surge is quick, sometimes only one day and if you don't test on that day, you could have missed it for the month. So you need to ensure that you test for at least five days before your suspected surge/ovulation. This can be a pricy item on your monthly budget.

Everything I wish I had Known Before Starting My Fertility Treatments

- The tests are all different. What works for one woman might not work at all for another. Personally, only the cheap paper strips work (very well) for me and I get very sporadic and unreliable readings from the digital ones. Because of this, you need to spend a few months and extra money using several tests at the same time as you try to work out which ones work best for you.

- An LH surge does NOT mean that you have definitely ovulated. Sometimes an egg doesn't emerge from its follicle and sometimes the body prepares itself for ovulation and then malfunctions and it doesn't happen that month. Only medical tests can prove whether you have actually ovulated.

- An LH surge kit or OPK will probably NOT work if you have PCOS, due to already raised LH levels. Some women swear by them but they are often unreliable for the majority of women.

## SALIVA-BASED FERTILITY TESTS

Why?

Before women ovulate, they not only have an LH surge, but they also have an oestrogen surge.

The oestrogen surge usually happens before the LH surge, so it acts as a type of pre-pre-ovulation warning.

At different times of the month when our oestrogen levels fluctuate, we can see what's happening in our bodies by looking at our saliva under a microscope.

As the oestrogen rises, your saliva will form ferning patterns — literally, your saliva will look like the leaves of a fern and this ferning is what signals that an LH surge and subsequent ovulation is on the way.

Again, there is a range of saliva-based tests on the market, all similarly priced. Shop around online or at pharmacies, read the reviews and see what seems like a good fit for you.

How?

As this bit of kit is reusable, you can start testing it out as soon as you get it. Once you've got the hang of it, I would say to start testing daily from around Cycle Day 10.

- Keep your microscope next to your bed for easy access so that you can test when you wake up. The test doesn't need to be done before getting out of bed, but it must be done before eating, drinking or brushing your teeth.

- Make sure you clean your microscope with a soft cloth (like those used for glasses) every time before using it again. Do not run the microscope under a tap (I learnt the hard way!) or even wet it with anything but your own saliva. I found for my best results, I licked the glass slide a few times. If you try to put a drop of saliva on the glass then it either doesn't dry or it clumps and doesn't give a reading.

- Leave the slide that you have just licked for at least 20 minutes – longer if you can – before attempting to press the light and look through the magnifying lens. The device will have an LED light to help you see.

- When your oestrogen is low, your saliva will look like bubbles, something like blisters. As your oestrogen rises, it will begin to form ferns (just like the plant) and when your oestrogen is at its peak level, all you will see are ferning patterns. It will be unmistakable. This tells you that your LH surge is imminent and you need to have intercourse.

## My Positive Points on Saliva Tests:

- Reasonably priced for something that you use again and again at no additional cost.
- Because it is reusable, you can use it every day of the month if you wanted without worrying about the cost.
- It's interesting (even exciting) to see how your body works and how something like saliva can tell you what's happening with your hormones and going to happen in your ovaries.
- It's a great pre-warning safety device to make sure that you don't miss your LH surge.
- It's small and discreet – the size of a lipstick.

## My negative points on Saliva Tests:

- The saliva can take a long time to dry, which is a little inconvenient if you are busy and can't wait for it to dry.
- When you first start using it, in spite of checking out many illustrations, you don't know what you are looking at and you keep wondering whether you are missing it – until you do see it and realise that it's so obvious you can't miss it.
- Some women just don't fern but you won't know that until you try.

- Factors like eating, drinking, smoking, brushing your teeth and even the way you put the saliva onto the slide can affect the accuracy of the reading.

## SPERM-FRIENDLY LUBRICANT

Why?

Laboratory tests have proven that most lubricants are toxic to sperm. I know that you're thinking 'So what? We don't need any lubricants.' Yes, I'm sure you don't – now – but give it some time of robotic intercourse for 10 days straight because you have to on those days to stand a chance of conceiving. After a while, romantic and passionate thoughts are pushed out by a rotation of baby-making thoughts – 'Will this be our time? I hope all those ovulation predictors were correct. Is my cervix open enough? Am I positioned at just the right angle for the swimmers to race their way up the cervix? And so on and so on.

*\*\*Something to note at this point, is that water and saliva also damage sperm and neither of these should be used during your most fertile days when trying to conceive!\*\* Something I only found out about a few months ago - this info would surely have been helpful about 12 years ago!*

"Hello Pre-Seed." This lubricant is clinically tested to not only be fertility-friendly, but to support conception by mimicking a woman's natural fertile fluids.

With all this said though, please remember that nothing is guaranteed. There are women who swear by Pre-Seed and are convinced that the Pre-Seed helped them to conceive and there are others who have not had any results from using it.

How?

- The tube comes with (single-use) applicators, which you attach to the top of the tube after opening, squeeze out the desired amount (2 to 3g are recommended), then insert as close to the cervix as you can. **\*Finding your cervix is a lesson in itself. Visit Fertility Nurse, Kate Davies' website, http://yourfertilityjourney.com for advice!\***

- Wait about 15 minutes, and then do the baby dance (BD) in other words, have intercourse.

**My Positive Points on Sperm-Friendly Lubricant:**

- All of the clinical reasons mentioned-above.
- It feels natural and non-sticky.
- No irritating side effects.
- Knowing that it's helping toward my conception goal, leaves me far more relaxed to enjoy working toward that goal.

**My negative points on Sperm-Friendly Lubricant:**

- It can dampen the already strained romantic mood when you need to administer an applicator measured out with lubricant, especially when you have to wait for time.

- The advised amount can sometimes feel like so much that you can't actually feel anything else, making the baby making process even more clinical.

- It could get pricy, depending on how much and how many times you decide to use it.

*The very lovely fertility expert, Kate Davies has recently done an in depth analysis of fertility apps and monitors on her blog, which you can read at http://yourfertilityjourney.com/fertility-apps-and-monitors and should prove extremely helpful if you are walking this road!*

# 2 INITIAL DOC VISITS & TESTS

Right, so we have tried all the previous-mentioned points for at least a few months and we are STILL NOT pregnant.

**What's next?**

Now, you need to visit your GP (general practitioner or family doctor) who will ask you a number of personal questions. From here on, there's no such thing as personal when dealing with the medical team.

Here is some of the info that will be required from you at **your first visit to your doctor regarding your fertility.**

Have the following info handy:

- Medical history – childhood to present.
- Medications you are taking.
- Length of time trying to conceive.
- How often you have sex.
- Whether either party has difficulties during sex.
- What kind of contraception you used and length of time since stopping it.
- Whether you drink and/or smoke and how much, or take any

illegal substances.

- Whether you are stressed for any reason.
- Your BMI (body mass index).

**Checklist for His & Hers Fertility Tests**

**His**:

# Full Semen Analysis

Volume – the number of sperm.

Normal: More than 2 millimetres (although too much could mean that the sperm are too diluted).

Density – the number of sperm.

Normal: 20 million to over 200 million.

Motility – the movement of the sperm.

Normal: More than 50% of the sperm must move adequately. They are rated on a scale from 0 to 4, with 4 being good movement.

Morphology – the shape of the sperm.

Normal: More than 50% of the sperm are normally shaped. Deformities can be present in the heads, bodies, tails or they can be too immature to fertilise an egg.

## HIV Blood test

## Hepatitis B & C

## Notes:

Sperm are always changing and sperm tests can read differently from month to month – therefore it is always best to do around 3 semen analyses over the course of two to three months so that an average can be taken, as it takes 2 to 3 months to regenerate sperm in the testes.

Alcohol, caffeine, tobacco, recreational drugs, herbal remedies such as St. John's Wort and stress all affect the sperm immediately and significantly.

Normazoospermia means normal sperm.

Teratozoospermia means deformed sperm.

Overheating, smoking, high BMI, alcohol, recreational drugs, wireless technology and tight clothing all affect the quality of sperm.

DHA found in Omega 3 fatty acids, Vitamin C, Zinc, Magnesium, Selenium, folic acid and Vitamin B12 are all essential for creating healthy sperm.

## Hers:

## Thyroid Function Blood Tests

Both an over-active and an underactive thyroid can prevent ovulation. Because the thyroid has an auto-immune function, it is believed to play an important role in fertilisation, implantation and fetal development and is linked to reproductive auto-immune issues, such as elevated anti-bodies. If your test proves that you have a thyroid malfunction, then your doctor will refer you to an endocrinologist who will put you on medication to balance your thyroid.

## Day 21 Blood Test to check your progesterone

This test is done on Cycle Day 21 hence the nickname. It is worked out on an average 28-day cycle, but if your cycle is longer, the day would be adjusted. If your progesterone level is low, it suggests that you did not (and perhaps do not) ovulate.

## Day 3 Blood Test to check your FSH, LH and E2

This test is done on Cycle Day 3.

The follicle stimulating hormone (FSH) check can be done to evaluate Polycystic Ovary Syndrome (PCOS), ovarian cysts and irregular bleeding.

High levels of FSH indicate low ovarian reserve (decrease in the number of eggs which can result in an insufficient number of eggs to ensure a reasonable chance of pregnancy), meaning both the quality and quantity are low.

High levels of the luteinizing hormone (LH) can indicate PCOS, ovarian failure and a number other disorders.

Estradiol (E2) is the most important form of oestrogen and cross-checks the FSH. If the FSH level is normal and the E2 level is elevated, it

could mean that the elevated E2 level is actually suppressing the FSH level to appear normal but in reality is high.

## Notes:

There is a new test that measures the anti-mullerian hormone (AMH) (ovarian reserve) which can be done at any day in your cycle and is apparently more reliable than the old-style tests. If your AMH levels are low, it is predicted that you will respond poorly to drugs in stimulated IVF.

## Chlamydia, PID (pelvic inflammatory disease) or any other sexually transmitted diseases

If left untreated, these can contribute to infertility. These tests are usually done with either a urine sample or swabs taken from the vagina or cervix area. Should you test positive for one of these, a course of antibiotics will be prescribed.

## Test to check for Rubella anti-bodies

Most of us got this vaccination as a child, but it can wear off after time. Contracting German Measles while pregnant can be fatal for the baby. If you no longer have the anti-bodies, you will be vaccinated again.

## HIV Blood Test
## Hepatitis B & C

## Haemoglobin & Scrum Ferritin Test

These tests are to check for iron deficiency anaemia, which is important for pregnancy as the baby will sap all your iron reserves in the first few months. If you are found to be deficient, your doctor will either advise you to get additional over-the-counter iron tablets or will prescribe stronger tablets or injections.

Sometimes deficiency could be due to lack of vitamin B12 and folate (very common in a vegan diet as vitamin B12 is only found in sufficient quantities in animal products).

## Hysterosalpinogram (HSG)

This is a type of X-ray taken of your uterus and fallopian tubes after a special dye has been injected.

This test is done to detect any blockage in the tubes.

It is an outpatient procedure that takes less than half an hour.

An HSG is the best method of seeing the shape of the cavity of the uterus. Abnormalities such as a septum (dividing wall) and fibroids can be picked up.

Generally this test is uncomfortable but not necessarily painful - however that feeling will differ from person to person.

## Laparoscopy (lap)

This is a (keyhole) surgical procedure performed under general anaesthetic, which will enable the medical team to see whether you have endometriosis (endo), cysts, scars or lesions and if so, to remove them.

An incision is made in your navel, through which the camera will be inserted. The surgeon will be able to check the outside of all your organs around your abdomen from your liver to your pelvis, including your uterus and ovaries. If any endo or cysts need to be removed, two tiny incisions will be made – one just above the pubic bone and the other just above the hip bone.

Your tubes will be checked at the same time (combining an HSG above).

The surgery itself takes around 2-3 hours, depending on how much work needs to be done, and you could stay overnight in hospital. The recovery time is dependent on each individual but the average time for recovery when endo or tubes have been removed, seems to be about 10 days before a slower version of your normal routine can continue and another 10 days before more rigorous activities can be taken up again.

This operation can be very pricey (I had mine done in the UK, which was just over £5,000), but it is a very important procedure to consider when you have had no success with conceiving for a number of years, as mild and moderate endo can ONLY be seen with a lap and not on an ultrasound, so you could miss it completely.

## Why is Endometriosis so important for fertility?

In simple terms, this is when parts of the endometrium (womb lining) grow outside of the womb and attach to other organs in the body. Instead of all the lining being shed each month during menstruation, some of it enters the pelvis through the fallopian tubes and begins to grow.

Endometriosis creates many chemical and immune imbalances within the body and a large percentage of women that are struggling with fertility have some form of it. This chemical reaction can affect fertility when trying naturally as well as when undergoing IVF treatments, as the body may be producing anti-embryo toxins from the endometriosis and therefore prevent implantation.

Endometriosis has four stages, categorised by location and depth of it:

Stage 1 – minimal

Stage 2 – mild

Stage 3 - moderate

Stage 4 – severe

Any of these stages can have a significant effect on fertility.

Right, so now you've done all the above testing and either it's come back with a problem which your medical doctor has addressed or there is no problem and therefore it's time to move on to a fertility specialist.

# 3 INITIAL CONSULTATION WITH A FERTILITY SPECIALIST

Both partners should attend the initial appointment as there will be many detailed questions asked and many forms to complete. You will find throughout your fertility journey that the same questions will be repeated by every medical professional involved. A good idea is to write down any questions you think of long before the meeting.

All your test results will be discussed with full explanations of what to expect from here on.

Things that might happen at your first meeting:

**Him:**

An additional semen analysis.

**Her:**

- Vaginal ultrasound
- Pap smear (if yours is not up to date. It is recommended that women

do a cervical smear every 3 years to check for cervical cancer).

- If you were diagnosed with PCOS you will most probably be prescribed Clomid for a certain amount of time before any other treatments start.
- If you do not go onto Clomid, then a treatment plan for either IUI or IVF will be discussed with prescribed medications and approximate timings.

# 4 TIPS FOR CHOOSING A FERTILITY CLINIC THAT IS RIGHT FOR YOU

- Get recommendations by family, friends or people in an IVF support group.

- Very importantly, check online reviews.

- Evaluate cost and if there are any special offers, what are the qualifying criteria?

- Do they have a proven track record?

- Is the location convenient for you?

- Do they offer any treatment specialities such as focused on over 40's, or specialise in donor eggs.

- What tests are available, especially when there has been recurring implantation failure or miscarriages?

- What techniques are available? Do they have the latest technology? What is the range of infertility remedies?

- Are they available for answering questions via telephone and email, especially after hours?

- What is your involvement in the decision making? You don't just want to be a puppet.

- What is the general turnaround time from beginning of treatment to transfer?

- If you're in the US, then check what procedures your health insurance covers.

- Will there be good communication between coordinator and doctor once you have gone for your first consultation?

- Do you get a genuine sense of the staff being your cheerleaders?

- Are they open on weekends and during holiday season?

- Clinic environment – is it calm, peaceful, welcoming, professional but friendly?

- Is there good teamwork throughout the clinic?

- Do they offer alternative treatments such as acupuncture?

- Are there any restrictions – BMI, married, single or gay couples, age, etc.?

- Are there any waiting lists and how long are they?


Going overseas for treatment...

How much time do you need off work?

How many visits do you need to make in that country?

What are the legalities, for example with regard to donor eggs?

What is their technology like?

What extra services can they offer?

Do they have an English coordinator or will language be a barrier?

What are others saying about this clinic?

Are there a number of good reviews, not only with regard to statistics but regarding communications, empathy and having their clients' best interests at heart? (See the resources page for international IVF coordinators in the UK and USA).

- Ask as many questions as you can possibly think of. Prepare beforehand and then contact them again after your initial visit if you think of something more – keep asking until you feel completely sure.
- Number your priorities.
- List everything you like about your short-listed clinics. Then list what you don't like and compare.
- Go with your gut instinct.
- Don't be afraid to change if you are not happy with them later on.

# 5 FERTILITY TOURISM

With fertility treatments becoming more popular, yet still very expensive, some countries around the world are cashing in on the thousands of couples desperate to create their families. These countries include, amongst others, Czech Republic, Greece, Cyprus and Spain.

These countries offer huge financial savings, state of the art technology, great customer service and many extras such as no waiting lists for donor eggs/embryos and anonymity for donor eggs/embryos.

Generally fertility treatment at clinics in these countries, with flights, accommodation and food & drink, is still cheaper than treatments in both the UK and the USA.

The most popular of these clinics (based on the many support groups that I am a member of) are the following:

**Czech Republic**

**Reprofit International, Brno (**http://www.reprofit.cz/en/reprofit-international**)**

**Reprogenesis, Brno** (http://www.reprogenesis.co.uk)

**Prague Fertility Centre, Prague**
(http://www.pragueivf.com/en/home)

**Gynem, Prague** (http://www.gynem.co.uk)

**Gest, Prague** (https://www.invitra.com/gest-ivf)

**Greece/Cypress**

Team Miracle (http://www.cyprusivfcentre.com/ivf-in-cyprus)

Serum (http://www.ivfserum.com)

**Spain**

Instituto Barnabeu (https://www.institutobernabeu.com/en)

Institut Marquez (http://institutomarques.com/en)

# 6 WHAT'S THE DIFFERENCE BETWEEN IUI AND IVF?

## INTRAUTERINE INSEMINATION (IUI)

- Used to treat premature ejaculation, erection difficulties and unexplained fertility.
- Most women take fertility drugs to stimulate additional egg production.
- Sperm is inserted into the womb at the time of ovulation using a catheter.
- Lower success rate than IVF.
- Significantly lower cost than IVF.

## INVITRO-FERTILISATION (IVF)

- Used to treat PCOS, blocked or absent fallopian tubes, endometriosis and unexplained infertilty.
- Women take infertility drugs to shut down and then stimulate the ovaries and ovulation.
- The eggs are collected under anaesthetic.
- The eggs and sperm are brought together to fertilise in the

laboratory.

- The resulting embryo is transferred to the womb using a catheter.

## A STANDARD FRESH IVF PROTOCOL (LONG PROTOCOL)

1 Down Regulation

2 Stimulation

3 Trigger

4 Egg Collection

5 Fertilisation

6 Transfer

7 The 2-week-wait

8 Pregnancy Test

Let's look at these in more detail:

### Down Regulation (down regging)

The first step in preparing for IVF is shutting down your ovaries. Essentially, you will be put into temporary, artificial menopause. And yes, most women will experience at least some of the menopausal symptoms that women going through natural menopause do.

Some of the side effects of down regging medication include:

- Night sweats
- Difficulty sleeping
- Hot flushes
- Moodiness
- Anger

- Headaches
- Reduced sex drive
- Heart palpitations
- Tiredness
- Joint stiffness, aches and pains

Down regging medication varies between countries, clinics and individual circumstances. It could be a nasal spray or injectables. Possible medication includes Synarel (also known as Nafarelin), Lupron and Buserelin (also known as Suprecur).

It usually begins on Cycle Day 21 and goes on for roughly 4 weeks (give or take for individual clinics/circumstances). In between you will have a withdrawal bleed and towards the end you will have an ultrasound to check that your ovaries have responded to the meds and have shut down.

## Stimulation

Once your ovaries are shut down, they will need be re-started and encouraged to grow as many, big egg follicles as they can. Possible injectable medication includes Gonal-F, Follitism, Bravelle, Menopur or Repronex.

The good news is that this medication alleviates the menopausal symptoms and you will start to feel better again almost immediately. The bad news, is that stimms also has its own side effects.

Some side effects of the stimming meds include:

- Extreme bloating around the ovaries
- Pain and swelling in the ovary area
- Ovarian Hyper Stimulation Syndrome (OHSS) – This is when a

woman's body over-responds to the medication causing fluid to build up in the abdomen and pelvis and could lead to blood clots. Doctors will monitor you very closely and if they see any possible signs of OHSS, they will reduce the amount of medication.

Stimms can be anything from 8 to 14 days depending on your individual body.

During this time there will be ultrasound scans every few days to check the status of your egg follicles. If they are responding well to the medication, they will grow between 1 and 2 mm a day. Sometimes the clinic will take blood tests to check your estradiol or oestrogen, which rises as your follicles grow.

Once your follicles are of a good size (between 16 and 21 mm), the clinic will arrange the best time for your trigger injection.

**Trigger**

This is an injection filled with the pregnancy hormone HSG and this tells the ovaries to ovulate and release all the egg follicles. The clinic will give you an exact date and time to administer the trigger.

**Egg Collection & Sperm Sample**

Egg collection takes place 36 hours after your trigger shot.

It can be done under general anaesthetic, heavy sedation or mild sedation with Valium.

The surgeon will use a catheter and fine needle to go in through the vagina and extract the eggs. The procedure takes around 20 minutes.

While you are undergoing egg collection, your man will be in his 'special' room providing a fresh sperm sample.

Eggs and sperm will be attended to further in the lab.

## A note on ICSI/PICSI & IMSI

Some couples will be offered one of the above. This will be part of your IVF protocol and not a separate procedure.

**ICSI** (Intracytoplasmic Sperm Injection): The embryologists will inject a single sperm directly into each egg to assist with the fertilisation process. This is often done when the number of sperm or the movement of the sperm is low or if fertilisation has failed in past IVF cycles.

**PICSI** This technique is based on the concept of Hyaluronan binding, which is a material found in most parts of your body, including around the female egg. PICSI selects sperm based on how well they bind to the Hyaluronan around an egg (in nature the strongest and fittest will bind). PICSI itself is a petri dish coated with hyaluronan in which the sperm is placed. Those that bind to these hyaluronany segments or dots are the ones that are chosen for the ICSI procedure as they will be the best quality.

**IMSI** (Intracytoplasmic Morphologically Selected Sperm Injection): This involves assessing the sperm at a very high magnitude using an inverted microscope which is about 6000x magnification compared to normal ICSI which is 200x. Embryologists can see subtle sperm defects not visible with ICSI in the head as well as shape, size and motility abnormalities, which can then enable them to choose the best quality sperm for fertilisation.

A few hours after your collection, you will be free to go home and rest.

On this day you will begin another medication – progesterone, which could be an oil to inject, oral tablets or pessaries to insert rectally or vaginally. Brands include Cyclogest, Crinone, Utrogestan, Endometrin, Provera and Prometrium. Progesterone is needed to prepare the lining of your womb and make it all cushiony for your embryo/s to snuggle in and attach.

Egg collection is major surgery, so it's advisable to take it easy for a few days after if you can. Some women unfortunately have a hard time recovering and need bed rest for a few days to deal with the pain, nausea and general feeling of being unwell. If this is severe, then you possibly have a case of OHSS and you need to keep your clinic updated on your progress in case they need to hospitalise you and/or delay your embryo transfer.

**Notes:**

The clinic gives you an estimate of how many egg follicles (follies) they can see on the ultrasound. Sometimes, you will be presently surprised after egg collection to find that there were more follies than they first saw.

Sometimes egg follicles do not contain an egg, so the number of follicles does not necessarily equal the number of eggs collected.

Even when the egg follicles do contain an egg, it might not be mature enough to be fertilised.

Everybody wants to see a good number of eggs, but it is the quality that counts rather than the quantity. Do not be disheartened if you only have a few eggs. There have been stories of woman only having one egg at collection and that egg has become their child.

**Fertilisation**

Over the next 3 to 5 days, the fertilised embryos are watched closely by the lab. The day after egg collection, the lab will contact you with an update of how many eggs fertilised and their progress. The lab looks for the appropriate number of dividing cells, that the cells are even in size and that there is little or no fragmentation between cells.

**Embryo Grading:**

Each clinic has a unique system of grading their embryos, but here are a set of guidelines.

The embryos on day 2:

Grade 1 – 8 cells – no fragmentation

Grade 2 – 6 to 8 cells – less than 20% fragmentation

Grade 3 – cells are uneven in size and have more than 20% fragmentation

Grade 4 – no viable cells and more than 50% fragmentation

Depending on the progress of the embryos on day 2, the clinic will decide whether they think it's best to transfer them to your womb on day 3 (cleavage stage) or day 5 (blastocyst stage).

The embryologists want to choose the best possible embryo that is the most likely to develop into a healthy pregnancy. If the embryos are not making good progress by day 3, they prefer to transfer the embryo to the womb in the hope that its natural state will encourage good development.

If there is a frontrunner (or more than one) that is clearly developing well by day 3, the lab will continue to watch it until day 5 and then transfer the embryo to your womb on day 5 or sometimes even day 6.

The blastocysts themselves have their own coding system according to their further development.

**Blastocyst Coding:**

*Fully hatched blastocyst* – each embryo is encased in its own shell which it must hatch out of in order to attach itself to the womb lining and implant. This would be a top result.

*Hatching blastocyst* – the embryo has begun hatching from its shell

*Expanded blastocyst* – the embryo is fully formed but has not started hatching

*Early blastocyst* – the embryo is not fully formed and cell types are not distinguishable yet

*Day 5 Morula* – the embryo's development rate is slower than the other embryos and therefore difficult to know whether it will form into a blastocyst or degenerate before the blastocyst stage.

**Notes:**
There is always controversy about whether a day 3 or a day 5 embryo

transfer is better and which is more likely to result in a pregnancy. Some embryologists argue that day 3 is better because the embryo is back where it belongs in the body. Others argue that by waiting for day 5, the best possible embryos are put back and more of a chance for a pregnancy.

However, in reality an embryo is going to develop, attach and grow into a viable pregnancy regardless. There are some women who have had 7 IVF cycles with day 5 embryos and not been successful while others have been successful on their first IVF cycle with a day 3 embryo.

## Transfer

Embryo transfer is generally a simple procedure.

A catheter with your best embryo/s is inserted vaginally into your womb where the embryos are released to find a place to attach. For most people this is not painful at all and the most uncomfortable part is having a full bladder. A full bladder is requested so that it is easier to see the position of the womb.

There are some women who do suffer from obstructions in their uterus which does make transfer painful and difficult, but it's not the norm.

Some clinics will issue Valium to calm the body for transfer, especially if they suspect that it will be a difficult transfer. Sometimes mock transfers are done beforehand to check for obstructions.

The procedure will take around 15 minutes and then you can continue with your usual activities. Depending on the clinic you could also be asked to lie down for 30 to 60 minutes and occasionally be instructed to spend the rest of the day at home.

There is quite a bit of controversy with regard to the best advice to follow directly after your transfer and for the 2-week-wait. As with many things in IVF, as you will discover, clinics tend to give contradicting advice and you will probably be left completely confused and panicking about doing the wrong thing because women with other clinics have been told different things. Personally I would say, that if you have trusted your clinic enough to get this far with them, then forget what you hear from others and do what your own clinic tells you.

Everything I wish I had Known Before Starting My Fertility Treatments

**There are a few things that they seem to agree on though and these are:**

- Do whatever you can to eliminate stress. Stress is a danger to your body.

- Refrain from strenuous physical activities like Zumba. Rather change to walking and yoga.

- No bathing (shower only), no swimming, no douching or using a bidet or tampons in case of infections.

- No heavy lifting or straining which could make your uterus contract.

- No intercourse within the first few days at least, in case of infections.

- Keep the blood flowing to your uterus.

- Eat as if you are already pregnant, meaning no raw fish, meat must be cooked well, no mould-ripened cheeses such as Brie and goat's cheese, no paté, no raw or partially cooked eggs to avoid salmonella and any harmful bacteria like listeria.

- Do not change cat litter boxes. Their faeces contain a parasite that can cause an infection called toxoplasmosis which is very dangerous to an unborn baby and there are no symptoms to tell you that you have it.

**The 2-week-wait**

For 99% of women going through fertility challenges, especially IVF, this is hell on earth – the worst part of the entire IVF experience. This is the time between putting those embryos into your womb and finding out whether they have attached and formed a pregnancy.

Essentially you are now PUPO (pregnant until proven otherwise).

This is what's happening in your body at this time:

## 3 Day Transfer:

1 day post transfer – the embryo continues to grow and develop, changing into a morula

2 days post transfer – the cells of the morula continue to divide developing into a blastocyst

3 days post transfer – blastocyst begins to hatch out of shell

4 days post transfer – blastocyst continues to hatch out of its shell and it begins to attach to a site on the uterine lining

5 days post transfer – blastocyst attaches deeper into uterine lining and implantation begins

6 days post transfer – implantation process continues

7 days post transfer – implantation is complete – cells that will eventually become the placenta and fetus begin to develop

8 days post transfer – HCG begins to enter the blood stream

9 days post transfer – more HCG is produced as fetus develops

10 days post transfer – more HCG is produced as fetus develops

11 days post transfer – HCG levels are now high enough to be detected on HPT

## 5 Day Transfer:

1 day post transfer – blastocyst hatches out of shell

2 days post transfer – blastocyst attaches to a site on the uterine lining

3 days post transfer – implantation begins as the blastocyst begins to bury in the lining

Everything I wish I had Known Before Starting My Fertility Treatments

4 days post transfer – implantation process continues

5 days post transfer – implantation is complete – cells that will eventually become the placenta and fetus begin to develop

6 days post transfer – placenta cells begin to secrete HCG in the blood

7 days post transfer – more HCG is produced as fetus develops

8 days post transfer – more HCG is produced as fetus develops

9 days post transfer – HCG levels are now high enough to be detected on HPT

While you wait for your little embryos to do their thing, you need to keep yourself HAPPILY busy. Your mind will be on a rotation of these questions… *"Has it worked? Does that cramp mean that the embryo is attaching? I feel bloated, maybe that means I'm getting my period and it's failed? Should I pee on a stick (POAS) or wait for my official test day? On what day did others get their positive result?"*

There are hundreds of suggested activities on the internet by others who have been there to get your mind away from that kind of thinking and obsessing, but you need to adopt something that works for YOU. Use your interests, the things that light you up and give you joy and your personal stress busters to keep you calm, positive and happy during this time.

## MOST POPULAR 2-WEEK-WAIT ACTIVITIES THAT HAVE PROVEN HELPFUL:

- Meditation and Mindfulness practice
- Adult colouring-in books

- A craft – sewing, crochet, designing
- Keep a journal/diary or blog to get your feelings out on paper and see them from a different angle
- Read a good book or watch a TV series that will keep you captivated
- Walking & yoga
- Listen to music you love and hold your own karaoke in your living room
- Have a clean out of your cupboards and donate or sell things you no longer need/want
- Catch up with friends and steer the topic away from you and onto what's happening in their lives

**What should you NOT do?**

- Research on the internet!
- Compare every ache and flutter and headache with everyone else's ache and flutter and headache – firstly, EVERYONE IS DIFFERENT (one of the most important lessons to learn on this journey) and secondly, the medication loves to mess around with your head and mimic possible pregnancy symptoms, so you never know what might be real and what is just the medication.

**Pregnancy Test**

Most clinics will insist on a blood test called a beta test, however, there are a few clinics (especially in the UK) who only issue their patients with a home pregnancy test (HPT).

**What's the BETA all about?**

A beta test, also known as beta HCG (human chorionic gonadotropin), is a blood test that confirms pregnancy. This type of pregnancy test reports the level of hormone that is present in your system. If you are pregnant, even if you've gotten a negative HPT, then the blood test will pick up the hormone.

We all have a small level of this hormone in our systems at certain times in our cycle, which means that for us to be pregnant and sustain a pregnancy, the level must increase every 48 hours. Some women are concerned about the fact that their numbers start off low, but as long as they keep increasing, you're doing fine. It is also important to note, that your HCG levels will still rise if you are having an ectopic pregnancy. When the numbers decrease instead you are in danger of having a chemical pregnancy.

**Ectopic Pregnancy**

Ectopic means 'in the wrong place'.

This is when the embryo starts to develop outside of the womb, usually in the tubes but sometimes also the stomach. It can happen even in an IVF pregnancy when either the embryo has been placed too close to the opening of the tubes during transfer or sometimes for unknown reasons, the embryo will move to the tubes even when transferred in the correct place in the womb.

This type of pregnancy cannot be saved and moved to the womb – it needs to be terminated. If it is not discovered in time it may cause your tubes to burst and is life threatening to you. Your specialist will inject you with a drug called methotrexate which will force your pregnancy tissues to be reabsorbed by the body. You will bleed for a few weeks.

If an ectopic isn't discovered early on surgery may be needed to remove it, but this rarely happens during IVF due to early ultrasounds.

## Chemical Pregnancy

This is a very early miscarriage that happens within the first week or two of implantation. The embryo implanted in the uterus but could not hold on and develop.

It is very common amongst all women and often happens without women even realising that they were pregnant in the first place.

## D&C (Dilation & Curettage)

This is a procedure to remove tissues left behind in the uterus after a miscarriage, especially a missed-miscarriage (when the baby has died but is still attached to the uterus).

The doctor will open the cervix and use a surgical instrument called a curette to remove the tissue. These instruments can be sharp or a suction.

The procedure will be done under general anesthetic.

## ERPC (Evacuation of Retained Products of Conception)

This is a similar procedure to a D&C above, but it is a suction.

## If your test is a BFP (Big Fat Positive) – one of the most important abbreviations you will learn on this journey! – then:

Your beta will be checked every few days for a week or two to make sure that your levels are rising (only at clinics that do betas).

- You will have an early pregnancy ultrasound to make sure that it's not ectopic and that a fetal sac, pole and heartbeat can be seen. This is usually done around 6 weeks. It is difficult to see anything before that.

- Depending on the clinic, you could have an ultrasound every week until you are released to your regular GP. Some clinics release you as a regular patient as soon as a heartbeat is confirmed in the uterus.

- You will probably continue with your progesterone medication as well as any other medication you have been on specific to your situation until 12 weeks pregnant. Again, clinics differ on this.

## If your test is a BFN (big fat negative):

- You will be told to stop all your medication.

- You will be called in for a post IVF consultation to discuss what could have gone wrong and be advised on where to go from there.

## BASIC/ STANDARD FET (FROZEN EMBRYO TRANSFER)

When do we do an FET?

- If you developed OHSS after your egg collection, your clinic will advise you to freeze all your embryos until your body is well enough to transfer them.

- You could decide to do several fresh IVF cycles (egg collections) and 'bank' your eggs until you have a good number of eggs to

  transfer at a time that is convenient for you.

- If you are having extra testing on your embryos such as PGD, then you will have a frozen transfer.

- Sometimes when using donor eggs or donor embryos.

Protocols will differ between clinics, but a standard medicated FET will be as follows:

1  Waiting for Cycle Day 1 (first day of your period).

2  Shut down your ovaries with meds to prevent ovulation.

3  Begin taking estrogen to thicken your uterus lining – orally, vaginally or patches.

4  Ultrasound scan to confirm that your lining is thick enough (8-13 mm) and is triple layered.

5  If all good, then you will begin taking progesterone – vaginally or injectables.

6  Transfer as per a fresh IVF.

If not good, unfortunately your FET will most likely be cancelled this time round.

## Natural Cycle FET

This is an FET cycle with minimum drugs for those that usually ovulate regularly on their own.

The clinic will wait for you to ovulate naturally through LH Surge Tests at home and/or blood tests.

Once you have ovulated, you will be told when to start progesterone.

The clinic will confirm your exact date and time of transfer which will continue as standard.

# 7 EXTRA TOOLS IN THE IVF TOOLBOX

As technology advances, so does IVF and various accompanying techniques are being introduced to assist with sperm selection, fertilisation and implantation.

Trials and tests have showed a significant improvement in success rates using these techniques; however, as with everything that involves fertility treatments, nothing is a magic pill.

Some people that have been successful after using one or more of these extras will swear by them and be convinced it/they made all the difference, but others who have used them – sometimes repeatedly – have had no success.

We have already discussed ICSI, PICSI and IMSI but here is a checklist of other added extras you can enquire about and consider using:

## ASSISTED HATCHING

What is it?

Tiny holes are made in the shell of the embryo with acid, laser or other mechanical methods, to help it to hatch so that it can begin to attach to the wall of the uterus.

Why is it done?

In multiple implantation failures, it is believed that it could be due to the embryo's shell being too thick or hard and therefore it is unable to hatch on its own.

Who is it for?

Two or more failed IVF cycles, poor embryo quality, advanced maternal age (38+)

When it is performed?

In the laboratory when the embryos contain an average of 6 to 8 cells.

## EMBRYOSCOPE

What is it?

This is an incubator that maintains the necessary physiological conditions required by a living embryo while they are in the laboratory. It has a time-lapse camera that continuously captures images and records them as a video of the embryonic development.

Why is it done?

Traditional evaluation of embryos are made at specific time points – once or twice a day and embryologists don't want to risk taking them out of their incubator too often. The EmbryoScope is the incubator itself and because it continuously captures images, the embryos do not need to be taken out to be looked at. In this way more detailed analysis is gained which assists the embryologists in selecting the best possible embryos for transfer to the womb.

Who is it for?

Everybody. Keep in mind that this should be discussed early on and often the incubator has limited space so you will need to book it.

When it is performed?

In the laboratory when the embryos are fertilized.

## ENDOMETRIAL SCRATCH

What is it?

The lining of the uterus (the endometrium) is gently scratched with a catheter passed through the cervix.

Why is it done?

It is believed that scratching the uterine lining causes a 'repair' reaction in the womb which could help embryo implantation for two main reasons:

It seems that endometrial injury increases the production of white blood cells which secrete growth factors, hormones and chemicals that make the new lining more receptive to embryo implantation.

Scientists speculate that the genes within the endometrium which are responsible for implantation are not 'switched on' at the right time. Scratching may switch these genes on to prepare the womb for implantation.

Who is it for?

The procedure is usually recommended to women who have had one or more IVF cycles with implantation failure.

When is it performed?

Clinics all seem to have their own preferred times and information is conflicting.

How long does it take?

Around 15 minutes.

Is it painful?

That depends on each individual. For most women it will just be a sharp pain for a few seconds, while a few others feel it severely. It is recommended that you take some pain relief medication about half hour prior to the procedure.

After effects?

You could bleed a little after the procedure so take a sanitary towel with you, not a tampon as there could be risk of infection.

## EMBRYO GLUE

What is it?

This is a solution in which the embryos are soaked in just before transfer believed to assist implantation.

Why is it done?

It contains a high concentration of implantation promoting hyaluronan and recombinant human albumin. It is thought that the hyaluronan in EmbryoGlue helps the embryo to implant by increasing the adhesion of the embryo to the endometrium. It also contains all the nutrients and energy sources needed for optimal embryo development.

Who is it for?

All those undergoing a fresh transfer.

When it is performed?

The embryology team will soak the embryos in the EmbryoGlue just before transfer of a 5-day blastocyst.

## MACS (MAGNETIC-ACTIVATED CELL SORTING)

What is it?

In this technique the embryologists separate the healthy sperm from the sperm which have less possibility of survival.

Why is it done?

A high percentage of bad sperm can be taken out from the 'pack', helping embryologists to choose the healthiest sperm for microinjection.

Who is it for?

Couples with low sperm quality, repeated implantation failures and repeated miscarriages.

When is it performed?

In the laboratory after sperm has been collected.

## MESA (MICROSURGICAL EPIDIDYMAL SPERM ASPIRATION) OR TESE (TESTICULAR SPERM EXTRACTION)

What is it?

These are sperm retrieval techniques directly from the testes using a needle.

Why is it done?

To retrieve sperm for fertilising eggs in IVF when there is no sperm that can be used in ejaculation or if it is difficult/impossible to obtain sperm in the traditional way.

Who is it for?

Men with azoospermia, which means they either have no sperm in their ejaculation because there is a blockage in the route between the site of the testes and ejaculation or because there is a partial or complete failure in sperm production in the testes.

Often men who have a reverse vasectomy find that they will need one of these extraction methods.

When it is performed?

A 'test run' could be carried out before IVF to make sure that sperm production is occurring at all. If a suitable number of sperm is identified then they are often frozen for later use.

Alternatively, once sperm production has been confirmed then the procedure is repeated on the day of egg collection and the fresh sample used for ICSI. If there are additional suitable sperm, they can be frozen for future treatments.

How long does it take?

Depends on which method is used and the individual clinic's procedures. Some clinics operate under a general anaesthetic while others only a localised anaesthetic.

Is it painful?

That depends on each individual. Most men feel uncomfortable for a few days and have some minor bruising and swelling.

## PGD (PRE-IMPLANTATION GENETIC DIAGNOSIS)

What is it & why is it done?

This is a genetic test to screen embryos that are at risk of developing a serious genetic disorder. This testing can help embryologists select embryos that are unaffected by a specific genetic condition and more likely to result in a pregnancy. These healthy embryos are transferred to the uterus.

Who is it for?

- Couples who are at risk of having a child with a single gene disorder through inheritance.
- Fertile couples who have a known history of a genetic condition in their families.
- Advanced maternal age (35+).
- Repeated miscarriages.
- Repeated implantation failures.

- A prior pregnancy with a chromosome abnormality.
- Carriers of a recessive genetic disease such as cystic fibrosis.

When is it performed?

Testing on embryos can be done from Day 3 cleavage stage – embryos are placed under a powerful microscope and a tiny opening is made in the outer membrane holding the embryo together. Typically one cell is removed and the embryo is returned to the incubator.

When testing is done on a Day 5 or 6 blastocyst, multiple cells are safely taken from the embryo through the small hole that was made on Day 3.

How long does it take?

This will depend on the clinic and the lab used – typically around 6 weeks.

## PGS (PRE-IMPLANTATION GENETIC SCREENING)

What is it?

This test screens for numerical chromosomal abnormalities.

Why is it done?

Chromosomally normal embryos are the most likely to develop to term and become healthy babies. This test helps embryologists choose which embryos to transfer by analysing all 24 chromosome types.

Who is it for?

- Women over 35 years old.
- Repeated miscarriages of unknown cause.
- Repeated implantation failures.
- Men with low sperm concentration.
- Couples who have had a previous pregnancy with chromosomal abnormalities.

When is it performed?

As per PGD above.

How long does it take?

As per PGD above.

## OVARIAN DRILLING

What is it?

A surgical procedure to assist the ovaries to release an egg.

Why is it done?

Women with PCOS usually have ovaries with a thick outer layer due to higher testosterone.

Ovarian drilling breaks through the thick outer surface and lowers the testosterone so that the ovaries can be encouraged to release an egg every month and regulate menstrual cycles.

Who is it for?

Women with PCOS who have not responded to medication.

The Procedure

The surgery is done through a laparoscopy (key-hole surgery) under general anaesthetic and the ovaries will be treated with a laser or heat to destroy the testosterone.

# 8 ADDITIONAL BARRIERS TO PREGNANCY THAT YOU COULD TEST FOR

## ELEVATED NATURAL KILLER (NK) CELLS

We all have natural killer cells within us that attack and get rid of dangerous objects/disease that enters our bodies.

There is a school of science that believes the reason for many miscarriages and implantation failures could be from women who have elevated NK cells, meaning that the immune system is attacking the embryos within the uterus thinking they are dangerous foreign bodies and this leads to implantation failures and miscarriages.

This is a rather controversial subject and many clinics don't believe this to be true. However, there are women who swear that once diagnosed and treated, they were able to fall pregnant and deliver a baby.

## Getting tested for NK Cells

There are very few clinics that actually do the necessary uterine NK cells testing, although it is quickly gaining in popularity. Uterine NK cells are different to NK cells in the rest of the body, therefore a blood test will not suffice. Proper testing of uterine NK cells is similar to a smear test.

The most popular clinic for tests is in Chicago, run by a reproductive immunologist (RI) who specialises in NK cells. Many other clinics around the world send their patients' samples to the clinic in Chicago.

Testing is expensive and time consuming, although with more clinics coming on board, costs are decreasing.

## Treatment for NK Cells

- **Intralipid Infusions**

What is it?

This is a sterile fat emulsion made of soy oil, chicken egg yolk, glycerine and water, which is administered intravenously to mildly suppress the immune system. It is believed that intralipid infusions are able to change the immune cells in the uterine lining, making the environment in the uterus friendlier towards the embryo.

How is the treatment carried out?

Treatments are administered through a painless intravenous drip which takes between one and two hours. Infusions are usually done a week before transfer day, on transfer day and twice more during early pregnancy. Clinics will differ in protocols.

Costs?

In the UK these can average between £200 and £500 per infusion, depending on individual clinics.

- **IVIg (intravenous immunoglobulin)**

What is it?

It is a mixture of blood proteins (antibodies) made up by the immune system, which are extracted from donor blood and given to patients intravenously.

How is the treatment carried out?

These are administered through a drip of 40mg at a time a week before embryo transfer and another after a positive pregnancy test. Sometimes infusions are necessary every 3 or 4 weeks until the end of the first trimester.

Costs?

Average price range seems to be around £100 per gram, so by the end of your first trimester you could have paid over £10k!

- **Steroids**

Corticosteroids suppress the immune system responses and have anti-inflammatory properties which could help to 'calm' the womb in preparation for implantation.

The most popular steroid tablet is Prednisone or Prednisolone depending on what country you're in.

You will usually start taking these about 2 weeks before embryo transfer and continue through to the end of the first trimester.

In addition to the tablets, your clinic might also suggest a steroid injection on transfer day, such as Solumedrol.

- **Blood Thinners**

Clinics will also prescribe daily blood thinning injections (such as Clexane) with steroids to minimise the risk of blood clots. These are usually started on transfer day and continue until the end of the first trimester.

- **TNF (tumour necrosis factor) Blocking Agents**

TNF is a chemical produced by immune system cells, such as NK cells, which promotes inflammation and allows the immune system to attack the source of infections. Blockers are drugs used to stop the inflammation and weaken the immune system.

## MTHFR Gene Mutation (methylene-tetrahydrofolate reductase)

Put simply, this is an enzyme that converts the folate you eat into the active form (5-Methyltetrahydrofolate).

Folate is Vitamin B9 and is NOT the same as folic acid. (Folic acid is synthetic and is not found in nature. It must undergo various transformations to be utilised by the body.)

The Methyl group of genes are responsible for the following:

- Switching the many cells activities on and off.
- Turning genes, enzymes, neurotransmitters, tissue repair, inflammation and stress responses on and off.
- Reducing the ageing process.
- Detoxifying chemicals and helping to supply the body's most important anti-oxidant.
- Giving us our energy.

When you have a MTHFR gene mutation, all of the above functions are negatively affected, which in turn can have a negative effect on conceiving and having a healthy pregnancy. Impaired MTHFR function has multiple negative impacts on DNA synthesis and repair, embryonic development, neurotransmitter synthesis, and cardiovascular risk factors.

There are 34 MTHFR mutations while 2 are specifically tested for – MTHFR C677T and MTHFR A1298C.

Let's look at another way. If you have a MTHFR gene mutation then:

- You will find it more difficult to eliminate toxins from your body.

Everything I wish I had Known Before Starting My Fertility Treatments

- You might have elevated homocysteine levels – which means that you could be in danger of getting blood clots. If so, your clinic might recommend daily blood thinning injections from transfer day through to the end of your first trimester.
- Due to this gene mutation, the anti-stress dial in your body is turned right down which means that you are not as equipped as other people to deal with stressful situations and environments (hence prone to strokes and heart attacks if not careful!).
- You will probably be deficient in vitamins B1, B6 and B12, therefore a vegetarian diet is not advised as vitamin B12 can only be obtained from animal products.
- Artificial folic acid (in pill form and within food) and most over-the-counter vitamins are toxic to people with this mutation. Your body can also not respond to other nutrients and minerals you put into it therefore you could keep getting sick.

What's a Solution?

- Seek out a specialist that deals specifically with the MTHFR gene mutations. Not much is known about this gene in general medical circles and your standard doctor might not even have heard of its existence.
- Stop taking synthetic folic acid immediately and all over-the-counter vitamins and start taking a high dose of natural folate and methyl B12. These can be purchased on-line through Amazon or various specialty websites. There are also prescription medicines given as shots and nasal sprays.

- Minimise exposure to computers, cell phones, tablets, electronic toys, digital cameras and other electronic devices.
- Swap your toxic household products, cosmetics and toiletries to natural ones with as few chemicals as possible.
- Swap all your plastic containers for glass ones as there are many toxins in all forms of plastic (Bisphenol A).
- Filter all your water or better still drink natural spring water (with essential lithium) and plenty of it.
- Eat naturally detoxing foods such as artichokes, asparagus, cauliflower, broccoli, Brussels sprouts, peppers (red, yellow, orange and green), avocados, garlic and berries. Just remember to wash them well before eating!
- Stay away from genetically modified foods (GMO's).
- Eliminate stress from your day-to-day life, as stress uses up the methyl groups which you will already not have enough of due to the mutation. Stress will affect other systems such as the brain function and thyroid and cause degeneration. Exercise and meditation are great stress busters – keep at it daily.
- Research as much as you can, keep eliminating harmful substances and adding beneficial ones.

## ERA (Endometrial Receptivity Analysis)

This is a genetic test to check whether a woman's endometrium is ready to receive the fertilized embryo and initiate implantation. Recent studies suggest that women have a small implantation window and that window is not the same for every woman.

Women who have had multiple implantation failure with good quality embryos will benefit from this test as changing the transfer date by a few days could be just the tweak needed.

The test is done as a mock cycle the month before, with the same meds that would be used on the real cycle. The clinic will choose a transfer date and a biopsy of the lining will be taken on that date and sent to the lab.

Results take 2-4 weeks.

If the results come back as receptive, then nothing more needs to be done and transfer carries on as normal, meaning that there is no problem detected in the endometrium with the transfer date.

If the results come back as non-receptive, then testing needs to be repeated before a real cycle until a date can be found when the results become receptive. This could mean a few mock cycles to find the optimum date.

This test is very new and was developed in Spain so is therefore more popular in Europe. At time of writing, there is one clinic, Create Fertility, in the UK that offers this test. And I am not aware of any in America and Australia.

The biopsy is uncomfortable for some and painful for others – as with most procedures, it is very individual.

Prague Fertility Clinic offers something called ASET, whereby they will stagger the transfer of the embryos over different dates to give women whose ERA tests have been non-receptive a better chance of implantation.

# 9 DONOR EGGS & EMBRYOS

## Donor Eggs (DE)

Sadly, a woman is only born with a certain number of eggs to last her life time and not only do these numbers get used up quicker the older she gets, but they diminish in quality with every passing year.

The 'too old for own eggs statistics' (both for numbers and quality) vary between 27 and 38 and but most references will agree that by the time a woman reaches 40 there are all kinds of negative issues surrounding her own eggs.

That is not to say that there haven't been many women who have fallen pregnant naturally or using their own eggs with IVF but realistically, those are the exceptions.

Fortunately, technology has stepped in to enable women with low egg numbers, 'bad quality' eggs and those with premature menopause to still have a chance at getting pregnant, by using the healthy eggs of a young donor.

The legal rules, procedures and waiting times surrounding egg donation differ from country to country. It is important to research and gather as much information on egg donation in your country as you can before you decide on where you will commit your money, body, emotions and future.

As a small example of these differences, egg donation in the UK is gratuitous on the part of the donor and the law states that any child born from donor eggs is entitled to look up information on their donor when they reach 18 years old. In certain European countries such as the Czech Republic and Spain, donors are paid and remain always completely anonymous. In the United States, the legalities surrounding egg donation is complicated enough that a legal contract drafted by an attorney is required.

In some countries like Germany, egg donation is illegal.

## The Basic/General Procedure UK & Europe

- Finding the appropriate egg donor for you.

You could use someone that you know (under 35 usually), find someone on a national database or rely on the particular clinic's database (average age range between 18 and 27). Some clinics (especially in the UK) have long waiting lists, while many others in countries like Czech Republic have no waiting lists.

Specifics such as hair and eye colour, height and build, general education level is a standard but in the USA for example, more detailed characteristics sometimes with pictures can be requested.

- Every egg donor must undergo a full series of physical and psychological testing.
- You and your donor will begin to sync with each other's cycle.

- You will be given a drug to control your period. It is usual to use birth control pills (BCP's) for this but there are range of other meds that can be used.

- On day 1 of your period (at the manipulated time), you will begin meds to shut down your ovaries – pills, injections or nasal spray. During this time your donor will begin down regging.

- On Cycle Day 1 or 2, you will start taking estrogen to begin thickening you uterus lining  pills, patches or injections.

- On roughly Cycle Day 12, you and your donor will be scanned.

- You - to make sure that your ovaries are sleeping and that your lining has become not only thick, but shows a triple lining that is needed for embryo receptivity. On the day of your period, your lining should be around 3 mm. By transfer time, a lining between 8 and 13 mm is considered optimal. If your lining is not thick enough at this stage, your clinic will most probably increase your estrogen.

- Your donor - to check that her ovaries have been responding to the stimulation phase and are growing a number of good sized follicles.

- Assuming both your scans are satisfactory, your donor's egg collection will be carried out a few days later.

- At this time your partner will also give his sperm.

- You will begin taking progesterone – vaginal pessaries or intramuscular injection of progesterone oil- to make sure that your womb is nice and snug to receive the embryo.

- The rest should be as per an IVF using your own eggs.

**Donated Embryos**

Donated embryos are what it says on this tin… a healthy, young woman has donated her eggs and a healthy, young man has donated his sperm, which are then joined together in the lab to create embryos.

Generally the fertilised embryos are frozen in the clinic's bank waiting for a suitable host couple and the process follows a standard FET.

Again, each country has its own rules, protocols, waiting lists and costs. The USA has some of the strictest rules which need to be scrutinised by an attorney and these also differ between states. Another option is also available in the USA, which is Embryo Adoption rather than donation.

Embryo adoption follows the same procedure as adopting a child that's already born. The adopting family builds a relationship with the family giving over their embryos. They share pictures, correspondence, meet up in person and learn all they possibly can about each other.

**Surrogacy – varies greatly from country to country. Our beautiful twin boys were born via surrogate 20 July 2017 in Kiev, Ukraine. Check out my book,** *My Ukrainian Surrogacy Journey: A Personal Account of My Mission to Motherhood* **– also available on Amazon.**

# 10 125 VALUABLE TIPS FROM IVF VETERANS

REAL ladies who have lived and breathed this journey, especially to give YOU a helping hand…lovingly supplied by the wonderful Rachel Campbell of Sprout & Co (http://www.sproutandco.com.au ), Fertility Coach, Inspirational Speaker, Support Group Guide (https://www.facebook.com/groups/1410596069231916 ), Fertility Foodie and Friend to all.

*Please note these tips are by no means meant to be medical advice, just a collection of helpful tips and opinions from a bunch of IVF legends who've been there before.*

## WELLBEING TIPS

✓ Go with the flow because not everything goes as it's meant to. Appointments will run late, drugs may change, cycles will be cancelled. IVF is full of unexpected twists and turns. Flexibility is the key.

Everything I wish I had Known Before Starting My Fertility Treatments

- ✓ Take each day as it comes.
- ✓ Quality and quantity of sleep is vital. 8 hours a night minimum is a must. The drugs and hormones produced can make you feel nauseous and exhausted. Listen to your body and sleep when you are tired.
- ✓ Remember to embrace other happy things that life brings you while on your IVF journey. It's the little things that will get you through the tough times.
- ✓ Plan something to look forward to take your mind off your cycle. It's so hard not to get caught up with appointments, injections, retrievals and transfers. If you have something else to think about it can help.
- ✓ Support your IVF treatment with holistic approaches like acupuncture, kinesiology, fertility yoga, reflexology (before transfer) and massage to help ground you. Find professionals that specialise in fertility to ensure you are getting the best possible care.
- ✓ Take time out to ground yourself in nature or just go to your happy place.
- ✓ Be still and take the time to go within. Give yourself space to meditate and/or practice hypnotherapy. Both are very important to support your wellbeing, gain a sense of control over your feelings, and to help you feel connected. Meditation and yoga retreats are the ultimate act of self-love.
- ✓ Just Breathe.
- ✓ Celebrate each little milestone.
- ✓ IVF is your life but don't let it consume you. Plan other things, have an occasional treat. Don't let IVF stop you from living today.
- ✓ Take the time to stop and look at all the good in your life today, all

that you have to be grateful for. Fertility challenges are such a struggle, it sucks quite frankly, but life is happening now too. It can feel that so much is put on hold as treatments unfold, so it's very important to value life every day and notice the small and fab stuff.

✓ Treat yourself to a little TLC. I know it can be hard to splash out when you are forking out for expensive fertility treatment. But allow yourself a little treat during this time. Whether it's a massage, spa day, day out or a holiday. Give yourself something to look forward to – you are worth it.

✓ Soak your feet every night, or every other night in warm water (not too hot), sea salts and a few drops of lavender oil. Always ensure that you are using true organic essential oils rather than synthetic or fragrance oils. If you have a personal or family history of miscarriage or your have been told that your pregnancy may be in any way fragile, please seek advice from a professional aromatherapist before using any essential oils.

✓ Think happy thoughts, laugh a lot.

## CLINICS, PROTOCOLS & DOCTOR TIPS

✓ Be the CEO of your own body. Research the various protocols and talk to those that have been there and done it before. Inform yourself about your body, understand your blood work so that you can ask your doctor and nurse questions, query them on protocols and discuss your progress together.

✓ Do your own research into drugs, protocols, response etc. Get all your pre-IVF tests done to try to establish your fertility situation (that's you and your partner), and keep searching until you find some answers (often tests like MTHFR and natural killer cells can be done early for peace of mind). Don't rush into any old clinic; look around for the right place based on your specific needs.

✓ If you aren't happy with your doctor, find a new one. It's important to find a fertility specialist you resonate with and can talk to.

✓ Have all your questions answered by your nurse or doctor. No question is a silly one. If your doctor skips over or dismisses anything don't be afraid to ask again.

✓ If your cycle is unsuccessful go back to your fertility specialist and ask about adding to and changing your protocol.

✓ Ask questions of your clinic, but also balance that with trust that they know what they are doing (don't go in blind and never take your eye off the game, you are 1 of so many patients and you need to ensure you are being looked after, mistakes are often made). It's really hard to give that control away when this is your life, but again, it's a balancing act.

✓ Listen to your doctor and assess their advice for your best interest. We sought the opinion of 2 doctors who both recommended fresh donor eggs. We got pregnant on our first try. I'm 43. My husband is 50.

✓ Pre-implantation genetic screening (PGS) and Pre-implantation Genetic Diagnosis (PGD) to test your embryos – this gives you a better chance of having a successful outcome. It may save you money and heartache in the long run.

## NEEDLES & DRUG TIPS

✓ Ice your injection site in whatever way works for you.

✓ Keep a coin in the freezer (disinfect it first). Before you inject, place the coin on the skin – the coldness will numb the skin. Swipe the skin quickly with an alcohol swab and inject that juicy goodness into your body…you'll barely feel the needle.

✓ The shots don't hurt as much as you think they will. Just do it.

✓ If you have a severe fear of needles, get a topical anesthetic cream to use before you inject.

✓ If you are needle phobic and will be alone make sure you have a "Battle Buddy" on Skype with you when you do your shots! They can guide and support you to inject.

✓ If you take your injections to work, bag or box each day for the week ahead. It helps when you are running out the door to just grab your pre-made bag. Buy a lunchbox and a couple of cold packs to keep your meds cool if you don't plan on being a total home-body during your shots phase.

✓ Just breathe. Don't get overwhelmed by the amount of drugs you are given. Trust and accept that this is exactly what your body needs to help you create your baby.

✓ Get your partner involved especially when injecting (as long as they don't have a fear of needles). I used to do it all alone and then blamed him for not getting involved but he didn't know what I wanted.

✓ Don't stand up when you're giving yourself injections, I nearly passed out. My blood pressure just *swooped* and suddenly I was sitting in the chair.

## YOUR CYCLE + EGGS, SWIMMERS + YOU TIPS

Everything I wish I had Known Before Starting My Fertility Treatments

- ✓ Learn all you can about egg and sperm quality and improving it. In hindsight I wish I had educated myself on how to improve egg and sperm quality.
- ✓ Look at your first cycle as a 'practice run' – its often a trial for your fertility specialist to see how your body reacts to the medications and the quantities prescribed, it's a learning curve for you both. Don't be surprised if it takes 1, 2, 10 or more cycles for success. If you really want this, be prepared to go again and again and again.
- ✓ #Have hopeful yet realistic expectations. The doctors don't always tell you how quickly numbers can dwindle and that is a very heartbreaking part of going through IVF.
- ✓ Take it one day at a time.
- ✓ Embryos can split. I wish I had prepared myself a bit more for that possibility.
- ✓ Phone your clinic if you have questions; that's what they are there for. Make sure you have your clinics emergency, after hour's number stored in your phone too.
- ✓ The realization of an unsuccessful cycle or miscarriage is harder than you initially expect it to be.
- ✓ Research every part of the IVF process in depth so that you can be an advocate for yourself and not just a passenger on a ride.
- ✓ Stay away from home pregnancy tests (HPT's). It's torturous and not always correct either way. I got a negative one day before my bloods and ended up being pregnant a few days later.
- ✓ Take it easy after your transfer. Be kind to yourself, gentle to your body and give your little embryo a chance to snuggle in.
- ✓ First 2 weeks will go-fast, but the 2-week wait will be very, very

slow.

✓ If you're a planner, make a plan for both outcomes after your cycle - a plan for relaxing and being productive if you have success but importantly, plan for an unsuccessful cycle which includes some play time, drinking and eating something not on your fertility diet e.g. wine and sushi or stay up all night… just do something fun and that you can't do if you get pregnant.

## NUTRITION + SUPPLEMENTATION TIPS

(Please consult your practitioner before taking any supplements)

✓ Start preparing your body, improving your eggs and sperm quality 3-4 months before your cycle by embarking on a pre-conception cleanse, implementing a natural fertility diet, cutting out cigarettes, caffeine, alcohol and recreational and prescription drugs (discuss with your doctor).

✓ Improve your chances of IVF with herbs, supplements and a natural fertility diet. Talk to your practitioner about fertility boosting supplements.

✓ Don't guess or take unqualified advice from others about supplements, herbs or diet – pay the money, see a qualified professional and get correct, tailored individual advice for your unique situation. Some things like Royal Jelly, Bee Pollen, MACA and really any herbs or supplements can cause adverse reactions, so ensure you are under proper professional care.

✓ Eat a natural fertility diet but with the odd little treat. Eat wholefoods – opt for fresh food, local, seasonal and organic (where possible) and cut out over processed and packaged food.

✓ Drink plenty of clean, filtered water and stay well-hydrated throughout.

✓ A high protein diet helped curb my Ovarian Hyper stimulation (OHSS). I had the onset of OHSS and eating a high protein diet helped tremendously with bringing the OHSS back down.

## EMOTIONAL TIPS

✓ You may cry more during your cycle than you thought possible. This is OK, let the tears flow, get your emotions out, feel the release. Look at the bigger picture and find something to laugh at.

✓ Don't carry the burden alone. Have someone to laugh and cry with.

✓ It's ok not to be hopeful and positive all the time; you're allowed to freak out. IVF is emotionally and mentally challenging and can be scary for some. One moment I'm my biggest cheerleader, the next moment I could be crying in the dark. Remember, so much of it is hormones. Be kind to yourself.

✓ It's ok to be selfish and take care of yourself ahead of others for a change. People who have not been through IVF have no idea what this roller coaster can be like. How many appointments there are, how much mental space it consumes. It's okay to say NO.

✓ IVF is not always a quick fix; it may be a long journey with many ups and downs. Cry when you need to, pick yourself up, dust yourself off and keep going.

✓ You may not be able to control your fertility, but you can manage the way you respond to the experience.

✓ Be patient. Don't expect things to happen overnight. It's a process with lots of bumps along the way.

✓ Be realistic about IVF. It's not always the silver bullet we start out believing it will be. Not everyone gets an IVF miracle baby. But if it comes to this, please know, there are many ways to grow your family.

✓ Don't be afraid to be honest, no one can tell you how you should feel. Find a counselor or fertility coach to support you, or talk to someone close.

✓ Plan something to look forward to take your mind off the cycle. It's so hard not to get caught up with appointments, injections, transfers pick-ups etc. Having something else to think about can help.

✓ I've learned to let so much bulls*&@t go. The things that used to bother me seem so petty in comparison to going through IVF. You won't have time to get wrapped up in the affairs of others; focus on your mental, emotional and physical health. Ignore all that other noise around you…it will only slow you down.

✓ #mustlearnpatience – I find the waiting game is so slow from submitting paperwork to waiting for transfer, and don't even get me started on the 2-week wait. Don't watch the clock or it will do your head in. Find a hobby, get creative, learn something new.

✓ Have loads of patience and mental strength. IVF is an endurance test of what you can handle as part of the baby-making journey. A cycle can be a roller coaster ride of hope and disappointment but keep the faith that you will get there.

✓ Prepare yourself mentally, this could be by meditation, affirmations, yoga, coaching or whatever it is that you need to get into the right headspace for your cycle ahead. Always remember the highs are real highs and the lows are real lows.

✓ Don't compare your journey to anyone else. *Comparitonitis* can dampen your spirit and takes you off course from your own journey.

✓ Keep a journal to write things down and express yourself. If you don't feel like talking things through, this is a beautiful way to process and heal.

## BODY TIPS

✓ Get some comfy stretchy pants and maxi skirts because you will be bloated, constipated, have tender ovaries and wearing tight fitting pants will be like torture (even if you can zip them up).

✓ Your body is not broken, it is not evil, and it is not bad. Go easy on it, shower it with love and in time good things will happen.

✓ If you are doing IVF on the quiet and are a bruiser, buy some tops that cover the inner arms for blood tests. It's hard to hide that you're having that many blood tests. And try not to feel like an IVF patient.

✓ Nurture yourself through your cycle with gentle exercise – walking, yoga and breathing exercise are best.

✓ Just be in your physical body. Sit in the parks, on the beach, in nature, read, meditate, get lost in the sunrise. Take time to just be.

## RELATIONSHIP TIPS

✓ Communication with your partner is a must. Mutual compassion between you is very important. Fertility challenges will try as hard as they can to rip you apart, but if you stick together, grow and support each other, you will come through the other side stronger than ever.

✓ Really talk to your partner. Care for each other. Tell your partner how to support you and ask him/her what they can do to support you. If you need a hug ask for a hug. Don't expect him/her to know. Everyone copes in different ways and needs different things.

✓ Remember you aren't the only one going through IVF, your partner is as well. If you feel inadequate chances are they do too. Love them and be a team together to win.

✓ Have IVF free dates with your partner. I think about IVF and wanting a baby most days. But we try and have a date night at least once a month where we talk about everything but IVF.

✓ It's easy to crumble, get off track and lose each other in this journey. Take the steps to ensure this doesn't happen to you. Counselling or Fertility Coaching can be a godsend.

✓ Look after your relationship with your partner. My husband and I have realised, that during our first round we forgot about our marriage and how lucky we were to have each other. Plan few date nights, go for walks, and watch a movie. Just be together and take care of each other's hearts.

✓ Pray with your partner and talk to your embaby, it makes for a wonderful connection.

✓ Before all the emotions, ups and downs, trials, fails, and bumps in the road, sit down with your significant other and write down why you are willing to go through whatever it takes to have a family. Make it serious, funny, optimistic, and meaningful. Keep this somewhere safe and when times get tough take it out and read. Use it to remind you yes it's hard, but yes, it's worth it.

## SUPPORT TIPS

- ✓ Talking it out helps a lot – find a Facebook group or support group to find others going through IVF, only they will understand how you are feeling and what you are going through. Don't keep your emotions locked up inside, it only festers & builds up making you feel worse.

- ✓ Budget a good fertility coach right from the beginning. I don't believe you can put a cost on mental and emotional health, both of which are extremely challenged on this journey. My hubby loves the lady I have been working with because he cannot believe the difference in me after coaching compared to before coaching. Many ladies view this as an unnecessary expense on top of the already crazy cost of IVF and all that goes with it, but I firmly believe it is essential. I'm not a coach or any service provider so I'm not trying to sell anything here, I just know how my coach changed my life!

- ✓ Think carefully about who you tell and when. Think about the impact, positively and negatively, for you, as to who knows and when they know. You may just want quiet space to yourself, or feel exposed if people say the wrong thing. So protect yourself in advance. Nobody else is expected to tell you when they plan to conceive their child, and neither are you.

- ✓ Share your story in safe places, Facebook groups can be enormously reassuring and supportive, providing both emotional and practical support.

- ✓ If you don't 'feel right' seek help. Don't be afraid to seek professional help. Making that phone call to book an appointment with a counsellor or fertility coach is the hardest part.

✓ Find a good support network. My 1st round was hell as I kept everything to myself not wanting to burden family and friends. I fell into a deep dark hole and found it very hard to come out of it. I hate to admit it but it nearly cost me my relationship. It has taken me 2 years to get to the stage that I can give it another go. Remember your mental health ladies.

✓ Find a cycle buddy. Or reach out to someone that has been through IVF that is willing to be your cheerleader. Know that you are not alone and don't have to go on this rollercoaster by yourself.

✓ Decide before hand how open you want to be with your friends and family. If you have a partner discuss this together, so you are on the same page.

✓ IVF is not a shameful secret. Share with those you trust when you are ready.

✓ Take advantage of fertility counselling. Most clinics offer counselling as part of your cycle cost, so make sure you check this out. Also check if any other support services are offered through your clinic. My clinic offered group counselling and it was here I met some of my dearest girlfriends.

✓ Check out **www.resolve.org** - The (USA) National Infertility Association is a non-profit, charitable organization that works to improve the lives of women and men living with infertility

## PRACTICAL TIPS

✓ Be prepared to spend more money than you budgeted for.

✓ Check if your clinic offers a plan that gives you multiple cycles and consider taking it. Your first cycle might not work even if you're a great candidate for IVF. In round two they'll know how your body responds to the meds and they can tweak your cycle for a better result.

✓ Keep a diary of what you are taking / injecting daily & how you feel. Sometimes just writing it down on paper helps if you don't feel able to talk.

✓ Keep a list of your meds and any supplements you take somewhere handy so you can inform others if needed (e.g. other doctors, naturopath, etc).

✓ Check your public and private health care and know what it covers for both IVF and pregnancy. Check what level of insurance you have and when it kicks in.

✓ Create a spreadsheet or timetable on your phone for IVF reminders and important dates.

✓ Don't use Doctor Google – it's not your friend. Google has stressed me out more than it has helped.

✓ Take a photo of your protocol sheet and keep it on your phone. I found this helpful on days that my anxiety levels were through the roof with everything there was to remember.

## LIFESTYLE TIPS

✓ Don't put your life on hold while waiting for your miracle baby.

✓ Talk to your work manger and try to reduce any stressful

workloads and leave work at 5pm during your cycle.

✓ Put YOU first and everything else on the back burner until after your cycle.

✓ Remember to get on with living your life NOW, plan trips and weekends away with your partner and girlfriends.

✓ Don't try and do too much or be 'normal' during IVF. This process is so hard, very few people get it and sometimes it's best to just step back and hibernate. This includes avoiding baby showers, pregnant women and censor your FB feed if it's too hard to deal with.

✓ Breathe & pray, take as much time off work as you need to prepare or while going through it all. Never feel guilty or ashamed of your journey, because it's one that only makes you stronger.

✓ You do not have to be superwoman! Lots of people get pregnant in various and exceptional circumstances, so give yourself a list of 'Do's' rather than 'do not's', life is about balance, not extremes. Give yourself manageable lifestyle routines to aid your fertility.

## INSPIRATIONAL TIPS

✓ Never give up (if you still feel the need to keep going).

✓ Smile often.

✓ Be kind and gentle to yourself.

✓ Knowledge is power.

✓ It all comes down to mental strength, hope and support.

✓ Be kind to yourself, give yourself little rewards for just getting

through a tough day or painful procedure.

Everything I wish I had Known Before Starting My Fertility Treatments

- ✓ Explore positive affirmations and keep the ones that work for you so you can look at them anytime; I have an album of positive affirmations. Place them around your house, store them in your phone, record them and listen to them.

- ✓ Don't take it all too seriously. Live life outside of your fertility race. It can be harder said than done but do try and keep the balance.

- ✓ Carry and hold crystals. They truly are like a best friend during this time. They help with the stress and work behind the scenes of what goes on with IVF.

- ✓ I took a different attitude with my last cycle that I wish I adopted on my first round – don't be so 'serious'! Still have fun with your partner, laugh with your friends and try to relax (the hardest thing in the world) and enjoy the ride.

- ✓ Read 'the secret' and believe – Get a self-hypnosis fertility CD and listen to it at bedtime.

- ✓ Be the master of your own destiny. There are a lot of things out of our control when it comes to fertility, but we can still make decisions around what we are prepared to do and how long we are prepared to wait. Doctors work by statistics, friends give advice based on their own experiences, but everyone is different. So if something doesn't feel right to you or you're not prepared to wait/do something, then go with your gut and don't be afraid to get a second opinion.

- ✓ Don't rush – take your time, listen to your gut, don't do something until you are ready. Even if your clock feels like it's ticking very loudly, make sure you come back to your heart and do what's best for you.

- ✓ Don't punish yourself: infertility is a physical thing, it's NOT a punishment or your fault - it just happens that way (people who have done bad things in life have babies all the time, so infertility is NOT a punishment).

✓ This experience will pass. Through it you will learn so much and your life will be enriched as a result. It can feel like it's stripping you back, but actually if you choose to work with it, then you can use it to make you stronger. Remember, something as beautiful and magical as a rainbow is the result of a rainy day.

✓ Any person who experiences IVF is incredible. You're incredible. Be proud of who you are and what you are doing.

✓ There are many ways to become a parent in this world – donor eggs, donor sperm, adoption, gestational carrier, step parent, etc. Everyone's journey is a little different. I was in a situation a few years ago that made me identify what was most important to me — and that was being a parent…even if it meant not having a biological connection or carrying the baby myself. That was way before I knew I would have fertility problems but it has helped during this process.

✓ Faith, Hope, Love.

✓ Don't become an IVF patient; instead you are someone going through IVF. Otherwise you will lose yourself. Remember this is your journey. It's so easy to compare yourself to what others are going through, but at the end of the day this is your path, and your path is unique to you.

✓ Self Love First. Look after yourself, nourish and nurture yourself.

# 11 FERTILITY SUPPORT GROUPS

There is no easy way to put this. Trying to conceive when you are going through fertility challenges can be dark, lonely, depressing and frustrating. Your family and friends, if you choose to tell them that you are doing fertility treatments, will try their best to be there for you. However, unless they have been on this road themselves, they will not understand your pain. They will not be able to offer you the support and comfort you need in the way that you need it.

The world of fertility challenges has its own language that only other members of that world can understand.

Fertility challenges has torn the strongest couples apart, has destroyed friendships, has put the once happiest of women on heavy anti-depressant medication, and has created pariahs in a society that places such importance on family and children.

Therefore, it is advisable to join a good support group where you can vent, cry, voice your fears, feel uplifted and get advice from those who have been there. There are many on-line support groups with new ones coming

up every day and it is important to find one where you feel most comfortable being a member of.

Below are a number of Facebook fertility groups that I have personally been a member of:

**Circle & Bloom Infertility Support Circle:** This group nurtured, matured and inspired me to be strong and courageous on this journey. Filled with a bunch of amazing ladies who emit love and care for everyone. This is a secret group - which means that only members of this group know that it even exists. In order to join, you will first need to join the general Circle & Bloom Facebook page which can be found at **https://www.facebook.com/CircleBloom**

**Coping with Infertility & Miscarriages:** Run by the very sweet, Samantha Rid, this group is an exchange of positive energy to help each other to become smarter and happier within this community. Here there are a mix of ladies trying to conceive naturally, through IUI, IVF, using donor eggs and surrogacy **https://www.facebook.com/groups/145592742511010**

**The Fertile Mindset Support Hub** is a place where you can go to for emotional healing, to reduce stress and to tap into your own strength to improve all aspects of your life. And by tap, I literally mean tap! The lovely lady who runs this group is Sarah Holland, EFT/Tapping expert (further details on the Resource page), who will guide you through the tapping process with video, audio, her book and she is always there to answer your

questions. Her closed group can be found at
**https://www.facebook.com/groups/FMsupporthub**

**Fertility Mindfulness, Manifestation and Miracles:** Run by the one of the most beautiful souls in the fertility community, Elisabeth Manning, this group is a safe place to believe in miracles and empower your journey to motherhood, making it one of joy instead of difficulty
**https://www.facebook.com/groups/consciousconception**

**Fertility Friends + Chat Group (Sprout & Co.):** This group is run by the most amazing Rachel Campbell, fertility coach, writer, speaker, blogger and fertility foodie – A few of Rachel's recipes can be found in this book and further details on her coaching service can be found on the Resources Page. This group brings me peace, calm, love and serious soulful connection to a group of wonderful, brave, inspiring, beautiful women whom I have grown to love dearly. It is always my first stop when I need to be uplifted or grounded. This closed group can be found at
**https://www.facebook.com/groups/1410596069231916**

**IVF Abroad Support Network** provides valuable information for UK ladies wanting to find out about clinics in Europe. Plenty of helpful ladies with an always loving, supportive and accommodating Admin, Sarah Jack
**https://www.facebook.com/groups/503806893130283**

**IVF/DEIVF group for the over 40's** is exactly what it says....for those

ladies in their 40's who are going through fertility treatments. A super group of ladies who are great at giving support and swapping relevant

information. This closed group can be found at
**https://www.facebook.com/groups/1391803797803876**

**IVF Support Prague** is a dedicated group for those ladies who are thinking of doing their IVF treatments in Prague. This group has a bunch of amazing, loving and caring women who will celebrate or cry with you (depending on what you need) and will all help with additional information on clinics in Prague as well as the city itself. This closed group can be found at **https://www.facebook.com/groups/1688538354766436**

**Let's Talk Infertility**
**https://www.facebook.com/groups/156104904783925** is run by the lovely, Lynn Collins, author of Sperm Tales. Lynn has managed an infertility lab for over 12 years and worked daily with reproductive endocrinologists and fertility nurses. She is always on hand to answer any technical or general questions.

**Path to Your Fertile Self** is a new (closed) group started by my amazing and lovable friend, Stephanie Roth. Stephanie had her son at the age of 43 after struggling with infertility and she started the group to share her tips with other ladies in the same boat and provide support:
**https://www.facebook.com/groups/1225661274157275**

**Solving the Mystery of Your Fertility** is a closed group that focuses on listening to your body and mind to discover what it is that could be preventing your baby from coming in. The aim is to be as natural as possible and to really get to know yourself. This group can be found at
**https://www.facebook.com/groups/solvingthemystery** .

**The IVF Journey** is another favourite. It is run by the wonderful Monica Bivas, fertility coach (further details under the Resources Page) and inspiration to all women everywhere. This group is a positive and up-lifting group that features regular guests from tapping experts, to embryologists, and fertility dieticians who are available to answer all your questions regarding their specialty and provide tips and valuable advice. There are daily themes from relationships to fertility myth busters. This group is a must if you want to be part of an active community run by the sweetheart of the community. This closed group can be found at **https://www.facebook.com/groups/theivfjourney**

And Bianca's IVF News & Notes, which I started in 2013 when I started my first IVF cycle. It's filled with all sorts of info from blogs to fertility events and service providers – anything that I feel might be helpful on the fertility journey: **https://www.facebook.com/IVFNewsandNotes**

# 12 ALTERNATIVE TREATMENTS BELIEVED TO ASSIST FERTILITY

## ACUPUNCTURE

A good blood flow to the uterus is needed for implantation and embryo development. Acupuncture stimulates the nerve tissue under the skin and in the muscle tissue which gets the blood moving. It is good for all over body health and the Chinese use it regularly to treat every ailment.

Acupuncture is gaining more recognition as a beneficial treatment by many mainstream medical clinics, who are advising their patients to take a course of acupuncture alongside their own treatments. Some clinics have even employed their own acupuncturists to take care of their patients in-house.

Feedback from the ladies in my various online support groups, is that acupuncture has helped them to relax, increased their uterine lining, improved the quality of their eggs and might have been the key factor in obtaining their positive pregnancy tests at last.

It is important to find a practitioner that specialised in fertility and that can prescribe a customised course for you (recommended at least 3 months prior to embryo transfer).

## FERTILITY YOGA

We all know that yoga in general is beneficial for the entire body – oxygen, blood flow, energy, relaxation, meditation, de-stressing and so on.

Fertility yoga has all these benefits plus it appears that it has the extra emphasis of increasing blood flow and oxygen to the reproductive system while balancing hormones.

You can find instructional videos on YouTube.

## FERTILITY MASSAGE

This kind of massage is said to increase blood flow, oxygen and energy to the reproductive system.

## MEDITATION

This subject has filled many pages and books over the years. It originally started in the Eastern cultures but lately the West is realising how important it is for life in general and how many benefits meditation has.

There is scientific proof that meditation can physically change the structure of the brain for the better. It can heal all sorts of physical, mental and emotional diseases.

Every person regardless of their situation in life should be practising regular meditation. It's crazy not to!

There are a number of types of meditation – from Eastern cultural meditation practises (Buddhist, Taoist, Hindu, etc), to meditations to help you sleep, to help you de-stress and also meditations specifically centred around fertility.

The general process is the same – find undisturbed time and a space, get comfortable, shut the world out, focus on your breathing and on the situation you need help or clarity on, relax and visualise.

There are many free guided meditations on the internet – YouTube, Apple Store and individual sites. You really are spoilt for choice – these days you will find guided meditations everywhere you turn.

I have provided some of my favourite meditations under my Resources Page of this book.

# 13 FERTILITY FRIENDLY RECIPES

My lovely friend, Rachel Campbell from Sprout & Co. has very generously allowed me to include some of her most popular fertility-friendly recipes in this book for you to enjoy.

For more super delicious fertility-friendly recipes put together by Rachel in a gorgeous kitchen companion, entitled The Fertile Goddess Cookbook, visit **http://www.sproutandco.com.au/cookbook**

In her own words… *"(my eCookbook is) jam packed with over 40 easy to make fertility boosting recipes to nourish and support you on your fertility journey! Whilst food alone was never going to fix my fertility issues, eating right certainly helped create a healthier environment for conception and a solid base for my pregnancy."*

## GREEN MACHINE SMOOTHIE

A fertility-boosting nutritional breakfast or snack to be enjoyed any time.

Ingredients (make it organic)


2 cups of your chosen organic nut milk, coconut milk or coconut water

½ small avocado or ¼ large avocado

1/3 cup frozen mango

2 stalks of kale (leaves only)

Handful of coriander leaves (alternatively you can also use parsley for a more peppery taste)

1 teaspoon of supergreen powder

1 teaspoon of macadamia nut butter

½ teaspoon of vanilla bean powder

1 teaspoon of maca powder

1 teaspoon of bee pollen


Method

Blend all ingredients together. Add a dash of filtered water or more milk if your smoothie is too thick and blend again (this will depend on the size of your avocado). Then sip slowly and enjoy the nourishment entering your body.


## IVF GODDESS SALAD DELIGHT

Pomegranates have been looked upon as a symbol of fertility for thousands of years... think of all those ripe juicy seeds as your gorgeous growing follicles. This jumbo salad will have your ovaries singing a happy tune.

## SALAD Ingredients (make it organic)

1 mango diced

1 green capsicum cut into bite sized pieces

1 pomegranate

3 large handfuls of rocket leaves

1 handful of basil leaves

1 tablespoon of sunflower seeds

1 tablespoon of pumpkin seeds

1 tablespoon of bee pollen

## DRESSING Ingredients (make it organic)

¼ cup of olive oil

1 teaspoon of maca

dash of apple cider vinegar

juice of 1 lime

Himalayan rock salt and black pepper

## Method

Combine salad ingredients together into a bowl. Mix dressing ingredients in a cup and pour over salad. Give salad a gentle toss before serving.

## IVF GOLDEN ELIXIR (A.K.A. BONE BROTH)

Did you know organic bone broth is one of the best foods to consume during IVF? This golden elixir is full of good fats, protein & minerals to help keep your energy levels alight.

Ingredients (make it organic)

2 pounds / 1 kg or more of bones, the more the better (grass-fed lamb or beef, and organic chicken bones including necks and feet work best) – get these from your local butcher who often don't even charge for them.
2 splashes of apple cider vinegar (super important to draw out all the goodness)
2 bay leaves
1 large onion
 3-6 pieces of garlic (depending on their size)
filtered water
any veggie scraps from the past week
a sprig of rosemary, thyme or oregano

Method

Throw all the ingredients into your slow cooker - the larger your slow cooker the better. Fill your slow cooker to the top with filtered water. Turn onto a low setting for the next 12-24 hours. The opportunities are endless when cooking with broth. Use as you would any other stock, pour into a mug and sip, use a soup base or mix a tablespoon into your stir-fry.

## HOME-MADE CHOC-BANANA ICE BLOCKS

Perfect for the summertime and free of refined sugar.

Ingredients (make it organic)

4 dates
2 bananas

2-3 tablespoons of raw cocoa

1 tin of coconut cream 400mls

dash of pure vanilla powder or vanilla essence (optional)

2 teaspoons Maca powder (optional, but huge super-fertility food points)

Method

Blend all together in a high speed blender. Pour into ice-block moulds. Freeze for minimum of 4 hours. Pour hot water on the outside of the moulds until they break free and pop in the freezer.

## PALEO PANCAKES

The combination of coconut, almond, buckwheat and berries are a sweet taste sensation and they're super easy to toss together!

Ingredients (make it organic)

4 eggs

120mls of coconut milk (or milk of your choice)

pinch of ground vanilla bean powder

2 tablespoons of maple syrup, and extra to serve with

60 grams of almonds to make almond meal (or you can use store bought almond meal)

60 grams of buckwheat to make buckwheat flour (or you can use store bought buckwheat flour). Alternatively you can skip the buckwheat and just use another 40 grams of almond meal – that's 100 grams of almond meal in total.

2 teaspoons of baking powder

1/2 cup of arrowroot flour

pinch of sea salt

pinch of ground cinnamon

coconut oil for cooking

coconut butter/oil/paste to serve

fresh berries to serve

any other fruit you may like to serve (banana, peach, mango)

Method

In a bowl, whisk together the eggs until they are light and frothy. Mix in your choice of milk and maple syrup.

- Grind almonds and buckwheat in high-speed blender to a flour (if using store bought almond meal and buckwheat you can skip this step).

- Mix together the almond meal, buckwheat flour, vanilla bean powder, salt and cinnamon in another bowl.

- Add your dry ingredients to the egg mixture and mix through well.

- Place a dab of coconut oil into your frying pan and heat to medium heat. Use a tablespoon to scoop a couple of pancakes into your pan (I managed to fit 2). Cook for a few minutes on each side, until bubbles appear on the surface and the bottom browns. Flip and cook on other side until brown.

- Serve hot with coconut butter or oil, fresh berries and fruit and a dollop of maple syrup.

# 14 FUN FERTILITY FACTS OR FICTION

The following is not based on any scientific or medical fact and is merely something light-hearted that can be incorporated into your lifestyle to make the journey a little more soulful and a little less stressful. It's a matter of personal belief.

**Crystals (natural form of stone) Gemstones (modified for jewellery) linked to fertility**

For more information and a deeper understanding of crystals, visit Colours of the Goddess, in which Karen Humphries discusses how she can assist you with crystal healing, chakras & essential oils

**http://coloursofthegoddess.com/work-with-me/crystals**

For gemstone necklaces and bracelets visit

**http://monicabivas.com/en/fertility-jewelry**

**Amethyst**

Helps to heal personal losses & grief

**Aventurine**

Encourage pregnancy and enhance fertility

**Black Coral (One for the MEN)**

Helps boost MALE fertility

Relieves stress

**Blue Lace Agate**

Protects during time of vulnerability & grief

Angels, inspiration and miracles

**Carnelian**

Passion, energy and joy

Helps to balance the reproductive system

Renews vitality

Improved flow of life force energy via the blood

**Garnet**

Balances sexual energy and enhances libido

Manifestation of dreams

Hope & faith

Positive & calming emotions

**Hematite**

Balances body's energy, blood flow and circulation

Regeneration of tissue

**Jade**

Aids fertility and childbirth

**Moonstone**

Aligned with the moon, which is considered feminine energy

Long history of being linked to fertility & love

In some countries offered to women as a gift to ensure large families

Ensures good female reproductive health & cycles

Balances menstrual hormones

Strengthens the immune system

Calms anxiety

**Rose Quartz**

Positive romantic & sexual energy

Promotes pregnancy

Protects mother & baby

Feminine Energy

**Ruby Zoiste (Male & Female)**

Helps the male and female reproductive system, especially ovaries and testes

**Smoky Quartz**

Balances sexual energy

Increases fertility

Relieves stress & anxiety

**Unakite**

Aids the female reproductive system, pregnancy and childbirth

## CHAKRAS

These are our energy centres that move around our bodies. There are 7 main chakras, all responsible for a different part of the body and mind stimulus. When these energy fields are blocked, it could cause illness, physically, mentally or emotionally.

Crystals and gemstones are associated with chakras and in turn with us, as we are all energies connected to the earth.

It is believed that a chakra can be blocked through variety of reasons – could be something physical or emotional that happened as far back as in our childhoods. They can be cleansed through using crystals and stones, sound waves and meditation.

**The 2nd chakra – the sacral chakra (spleen) is associated with fertility** (the ovaries, testes, menstrual cycle and reproduction system). It can be found on the lower abdomen under the naval. It connects with the energy of the moon, the flow of water, the colour orange (sometimes very light blue or occasionally white).

Healing the Sacral Chakra:

*Gemstones*: Citrine, Carnelian, Orange Calcite and other orange stones and Moonstone

*Meditation*: as mentioned previously, see the Resources Page of this book for great links

*Foods*:  Oranges, melons, coconuts and cinnamon

*Essential Oils*:  Sandalwood, Patchouli, Orange, Rose, Ylang Ylang, Clary Sage, Rosewood, Jasmine and Orange Blossom (Neroli).

*Water*:  Relaxing outside near open water such as lakes, rivers, streams and the sea help to cleanse this chakra – put your feet in, swim or have a refreshing shower.

*Yoga Poses*:  Poses should focus on hip opening, be slow and relaxed (eg. Open Angle pose or Bound Angle pose). Again, many examples can be found on YouTube.

## OTHER (MYTHICAL) ITEMS RELATED TO FERTILITY

*Animals*: Turtles, Rabbits, Butterflies (new souls seeking life – represents our desire to embrace new life), Frog, Wild Boar, Elephants

*Flowers*:  The Lotus Flower, Hyacinth, Apple Blossom, Apple trees in bloom

*Feng Shui*:  Elephants (place a pair on either side of the bedroom door or one statue in the living room) – Single piece of hollow bamboo (place in the north of the bedroom) – red paper lanterns (hung on either side of the bed)

*Colours*:  Orange & Red

For even more fun fertility fact or fiction, visit

**http://yourfertilityjourney.com/forget-searching-for-the-storkthe-secret-is-in-the-peacock** and read my guest post on Fertility Specialist, Kate Davies' blog. Find out why you should be looking for a peacock right now and other Chinese fertility mythology.

# 15 TIPS FOR KEEPING THE JOY IN YOUR LIFE DURING FERTILITY TREATMENTS

Fertility Specialist, Kate Davies holds regular Q&A Sessions for members of her online support group, in which I was a guest discussing how we can keep sane and happy while dealing with the uglies of fertility challenges and treatments. The following is a summary of that discussion, gained from my own experience working with a phenomenal fertility coach, Rosanne Austin from (**http://www.frommaybetobaby.com**), who became my lifeline and helped to find my happy no matter what!

The first and most important thing I want to tell you is that YOU ARE NOT your fertility struggles. They are just a small percentage of who you are – in fact they are not even who you are. They are just something you are going through – an experience, one of many experiences that your life is made up of. YOU ARE NOT an infertility statistic.

This is what you are…YOU ARE a complex, fascinating, wonderful, loving, fun woman. YOU ARE MORE than your fertility struggles.

If the above statements are not yet part of your reality, then we need to make some adjustments to make those true to you.

## Summary

1 Blame – drop it.

2 Friends – be realistic

3 Choose a life independent of your fertility journey

- Separate goals

- Be happy not busy

- Be social

- Volunteer

4 Have a nourishing & strengthening routine

5 Be your own hero

6 Be careful who & what you let in

7 Life is not a quick fix

## Blame – drop it

Don't blame yourself, god, bad luck, fate, life, your body, etc for your situation – it's not anyone's fault – it just is. Life just is. Good and bad things happen to good and bad people. It's just life. Blame makes you angry and stressed. Not a good combo for trying to conceive. Blame makes you see the problem and not the solution.

Don't be angry and lash out at people who are pregnant, that have children or at people who ask you if you have children. It's not their fault

either, so stop blaming them by being angry, bitter and jealous.

Everything I wish I had Known Before Starting My Fertility Treatments

Stop blaming your body for letting you down. Rather look at the ways that your body has NOT let you down. You can walk, talk, see, hear and so much more…your body has not let you down.

## Friends – be realistic

- Don't be angry with your friends if they have pulled away from you or have not continuously checked up on you since you have been on the fertility challenge. Everyone is going through some kind of challenge of their own, don't be so hard on them. Women on a difficult fertility journey tend to become the most bitter, jealous, hateful, miserable, self-obsessed crazies. You might not realise it, but you are not a pleasure to be around – I know this, because I was one of those women. Have a serious thought about whether you would want to spend time with you. Look at yourself through others' eyes and it might shock you. When last were you a shoulder for your friends? When last did your conversations involve things other than yourself or trying to conceive? Can you blame your friends for pulling away?

- Sometimes, the reason we lose our friends is due to us pulling away from them simply because we become so down and lose all self-confidence and generally lose ourselves, to the point that we have isolated ourselves from everyone that cares. They have probably tried many times to draw you in and include you, but you have put up the barriers. Most likely if you go back to them right now, they will welcome you with love and open arms. Again, be gentle and kind – and yes they might not say the right things - not because they are mean but because they think what they are saying is helpful. Good friends will be sad to see you so sad and struggling and will feel helpless and not know what to say or how to make you feel better. Even the wrong things they say often comes from a place of love. Don't be so hard on them.

- Of course, sadly there are also those friends who turn out not to be very good friends. I have had those too. The ones that just wouldn't even try to understand what I was going through. The ones that didn't care whether they were being insensitive or not. The ones that were offended when I turned down invites to do things with them due to being so ill from the meds, or didn't go to a baby shower because I would break down uncontrollably, etc. As far as I'm concerned, those are not real friends at all. Those are the friends that I just let go of. This journey is stressful enough as it is, the last thing we need is for our friends to put extra pressure on us. Best to cut those particular people out of your life, but still be gentle and kind doing it. I would advise first to check through a) to c) above before you do that, to be clear on the situation.

**Choose a life independent of your fertility journey**

Have goals separate from trying to conceive. Just because you are not yet achieving the desired result in fertility, doesn't mean that you can't achieve success in other areas. The worst thing we can do is live from cycle to cycle – that's not living, that's just existing.

Set yourself regular fun and achievable goals. These must make you feel good when you accomplish them. It's no point in setting goals just

because … and that don't mean that much to you.

What are your interests? What have you always wanted to do? What makes you happy? What makes you smile? What makes the time go by without you realising it? What are some things that you could do all day or night just because you love to do them? Start working on those. It doesn't matter how big or small.

Start a blog, learn a different language, get out into nature for regular walks, join a sports club...there are so many things that you could do. Explore your own interests and do what you enjoy.

## Do the things that make you happy – not just busy

Being busy does nothing to your mind, body or soul. You don't need to keep 'busy'. Just do the things that you love and enjoy and that make you happy and feel good. Stress levels automatically reduce when you are happy. It's very difficult to be happy and stressed at the same time.

## Do something social regularly

Our online fertility support groups are great and good for us, but as we all know, too much of a good thing can be a bad thing. This is when we obsessively read every single post every minute of the day to the exclusion of everything else.

You also need to join groups that have nothing to do with fertility. Better still, get off the phone or computer and go and be social with people. Join the gym, do the classes and start talking to people. Join a bookclub. Volunteer at a charity. Have a regular movie night with friends and a date night with your partner.

## Do something for charity

Helping others – whether its people or animals – helps us to forget about our problems for a little while and makes us feel good. There are so many that are in need of our help somewhere.

**Put together your nourishing and strengthening routine**

Every week I make sure that I do the following things for my own well-being:

- ✓ Meditate (I do this daily)
- ✓ Light candles and burn essential oils – Orange Blossom, Neroli, Sandalwood and Clary Sage are a few of my favourites.
- ✓ Read something positive – bits from a book, an article, or something good that's come across my news feed  - A book I highly recommend is called *Light is the New Black* by Rebecca Campbell – it's one of my all time favourites – it will lift you up and empower you as a woman.
- ✓ Put on music and dance around the house like crazy!
- ✓ Play with my cats.
- ✓ Find something that will make me laugh – a film or TV program – anything involving animals doing funny things usually does it for me.
- ✓ Learn at least one new thing about any subject DAILY.
- ✓ Do something toward the short, medium and long-term goals I've set and evaluate my progress.
- ✓ Play my "I am my own hero" music playlist. Make your own playlists with music that gives you oomph and makes you feel powerful and happy!

**Be your own hero**

Also check out my Huffington Post entry on being your own hero

**http://www.huffingtonpost.com/entry/10-ways-to-be-your-own-hero_us_579b56e4e4b00e7e269f0d47**

Stop being a victim. Stop being just a survivor. Be a hero. Be YOUR hero. What qualities do you admire in your heroes? Be that! What would your hero do in any given situation?

Create your story. Create your adventures, create all sorts of dreams, endless possibilities and ways to bring happiness to your life no matter what. Don't just react to life. Act, be, go, do.

Create your alter ego – give her (or him) a name. What does she look like? What is her personality like? Always try to check in with her first and see what she would do…. Then act and think accordingly.

Use visualisation – see the picture clearly – see how you are going to overcome your obstacles.

Don't rely on other people to make you happy, to make things happen in your life, to drag you out of misery, you are perfectly capable to be that strength for yourself. You are everything that you need. Your treasure house is inside you.

Sit down and write out what a perfect day would be for you if both this fertility journey and children were not part of it. Be creative.

Who are the people in your life that already make you happy and who would you want to spend the perfect day with?

What are the things in your life now that already make you happy? What are the things that you have the power over to incorporate into your life – study, fun classes, new skills, travel, etc?

What does that perfect day feel like?

What can you do now to make that happen?

Most important – BE YOURSELF. Be the best self that you can be. Don't compare yourself or your life to others – if you do that, you will always be a second rate imposter. Let your uniqueness shine. If you allow yourself to be your true self then your world will automatically fall into place.

**Choose wisely who and what you let in**

Choose to surround yourself only with people and situations that will empower, inspire and encourage you. You must choose who and what you let into your life. If anyone drags you down it's your fault for allowing it to happen.

**Life is not a quick fix**

These tips are not to pass time. They are not a magic wand to get you a family. This is a permanent lifestyle revamp. You need to permanently change your outlook on life in order to have the best life no matter what.

If you want to feel happy – do things that make you feel happy on a daily basis.

If you want to feel stronger – do things that inspires that feeling every day.

**Now go out and rock this journey!**

**You've got this. You can do it.**

# 16 FERTILITY RESOURCES

**Acupuncturists and/or Traditional Chinese Medicine (TCM) Practitioners**

*Andrew Loosely* – Natural Fertility Expert

World Leading Chinese Medicine Fertility Expert, Author & Speaker

Website: **http://www.andrewloosely.com**

*Nicola Salmon* – Hedgehog Healing

Website: **http://hedgehoghealing.com/acupuncture**

Email: **nicola@hedgehoghealing.com**

Tel: +44 (0) 7817 244 762

**Blogs**

**Kari Bengston** - Infertile Midnight Baker -

https://infertilemidnightbaker.wordpress.com

Karen Humphries – Colours of the Goddess -
http://coloursofthegoddess.com/blog

Kate Davies – Your Fertility Journey -
http://yourfertilityjourney.com/category/blog

Katie Ryan – Fertility Mentor – www.katieryan.com.au

Lori Shandle-Fox - Laughing IS Conceivable -
http://laughingisconceivable.com

Monica Bivas IVF Coach - http://monicabivas.com/en/blog

Rachel Campbell – Sprout & Co. -
http://www.sproutandco.com.au/blog

Rosanne Austin - From Maybe to Baby -
https://www.frommaybetobaby.com/blog

Ruud Awakenings - http://www.ruudawakenings.com

Stephanie Roth - B Method - http://www.conceiveivf.com/blog/b-method

Where's My Stork – www.wheresmystork.com

Your Fertile Self - http://www.yourfertileself.com/blog

Xtraordinary Fertility -

http://www.xtraordinaryfertility.com/index.php/coaching/justsayin

**Books**

Alan E. Beer, MD – *Is Your Body Baby-Friendly? Unexplained infertility, miscarriage & IVF Failure – Explained*
Amazon: **http://a.co/asJsuXa**

Brigid Moss – *IVF: An Emotional Companion*
Amazon: **https://www.amazon.com/Ivf-Emotional-Companion-Brigid-Moss/dp/0007414331**

Karen Humphries – *The Awakening of the Divine Goddess Workbook*
Website: **http://coloursofthegoddess.com/work-with-me/workbooks**

Karen Humphries – *The Empowerment Guide for the Spirited Woman*
FREE on the website:
**http://coloursofthegoddess.com/meditation-mindfulness**

Lori Shahine, MD, FACOG – *Not Broken: An Approachable Guide to Miscarriage and Recurrent Pregnancy Loss*

**Available on Amazon**

Website: **lorashahine.com**

Lori Shahine, MD, FACOG with Stephanie Gianarelli, LAC, FABORM – *Planting the Seeds of Pregnancy: An Integrative Approach to Fertility Care*

**Available on Amazon**

Website: **Pacific NW Fertility and IVF Specialists**
**www.pnwfertility.com**


Lori Shandle-Fox – *Laughing IS Conceivable: One Woman's Extremely Funny Peek into the Extremely Unfunny World of Infertility*
Website: **http://laughingisconceivable.com**


Lynn M. Collins – *Sperm Tales: An Informative Guide Through the Challenges of Infertility*
Amazon: **http://a.co/cQNau2S**


Nicola Salmon – *Nurture Fertility Journal*
Website: **http://hedgehoghealing.com/shop**


Rachel Campbell – *The Fertile Goddess Cookbook*
Website: **http://www.sproutandco.com.au/cookbook**


Rachel McGrath – *Finding the Rainbow*
Website: **http://www.findingtherainbow.net**


Rebecca Fett – *It Starts with the Egg*
Website: **http://www.itstartswiththeegg.com**

Richard Mackney & Rosi Bray – *Get A Life: His & Hers Survival Guide to IVF*

Website: **http://www.ivfsurvivalguide.com**


**Coaches**


*Elizabeth Manning* – Fertile Living & Conscious Conception

Board of Advisors for Tedx, Master Certified Spirit Coach, American Fertility Association, Associate of Prenatal Psychology & Health

Birth yourself first: Create a thriving, fertile environment inside and out to enjoy the journey and birth your potential. This is a proven method to take your fertility to the next level. By understanding the interconnection of fertility and life itself - using the science of epigenetics, the power of Spirit, and healing subconscious blocks to optimize fertility while stepping into the best parent I know you want to be!


Explore Elisabeth's website for a sneak preview of her upcoming book and 2017 May Fertility retreat in Sonoma for private coaching with Elisabeth and being in a powerful group setting.

Online group coaching course coming in 2017! Get on the waiting list as soon as you can.

Website: **http://consciousconception.net**

Email: **elisabeth@consciousconception.net**


*Karen Humphries* – Colours of the Goddess

Women's wellness mentor to empower the modern spirited woman to embrace a life they love to live. Wellness for mind, body and spirt.

Website: **http://coloursofthegoddess.com**

**Kate Davies** – Your Fertility Journey

Equipping you with the tools you need to navigate your fertility journey.

Website: **http://yourfertilityjourney.com**

Email: **kate@yourfertilityjourney.com**

Tel: +44 (0) 773 9329785

**Kathy Rustell** – Well Conceived

Life & Mindfulness Coach

Website: **http://makestressworkforyou.com**

**Katie Ryan** – Fertility Mentor

Use the natural wisdom of your body to discover why you haven't conceived yet and what you can do about it.

Website: **www.katieryan.com.au**

**Monica Bivas** – Monica Bivas IVF Coach

The Journey with Love Program for your 2-week-wait and beyond

Website: **http://monicabivas.com/en/program-options**

Facebook coaching page:

**https://www.facebook.com/monicabivasIVFcoach**

**Nicola Salmon** – Hedgehog Healing

Supporting women who are struggling to get pregnant make the best decisions for their health & wellbeing.

Website: **http://hedgehoghealing.com**

Email: **nicola@hedgehoghealing.com**

Tel: +44 (0) 7817 244 762

### *Rachel Campbell* – Sprout & Co.

Assisting women with fertility wellness and nutrition and a support on the fertility rollercoaster from a personal, emotional and practical aspect.

Website: **www.sproutandco.com.au**

eCourse designed to sync with your IVF cycle to nurture your mind, body & spirit:

**http://www.sproutandco.com.au/ecourse**

Email: **rachel@sproutandco.com.au**

### *Renee Waggener* – Xtraordinary Fertility

Empowering women and couples to re-birth their fertility journey through meditations, personalized strategies, & certified coaching, turning heart ache and tears into peace and balance no matter the outcome.

Website: **www.xtraordinaryfertility.com**

Facebook: **https://www.facebook.com/xtraordinaryfertility**

Email: **renee@extraordinarylifecoach.com**

### *Rosanne Austin* – From Maybe to Baby

Fertility Journey Transformational Coach who helps women to overcome the fear and stress associated with the fertility journey, and be happy no matter what.

Website: **www.frommaybetobaby.com**

Email: **rosanne@maybetomaybe.com**

### *Sarah Holland* – Fertile Mindset

Combining EFT methods to reduce stress and deal with the emotional issues relating to your fertility journey.

Website: **http://www.fertilemindset.com**

Email: **sarah.fertilemindset@gmail.com**

Tel: +44 (0) 7981 231 392

*Stephanie Roth* – Your Fertile Self

Assisting women to take control of their bodies and creating the most fertile environment when trying for a baby.

Website: **http://www.yourfertileself.com**

Email: **Stephanie@yourfertileself.com**

Tel: +1 202-365-8012

**Tiffany Jo Baker** – 3x Surrogate, Speaker, Writer, Couples Life & Fertility Coach

Website: **https://www.tiffanyjobaker.com**

**EFT / Tapping**

*Sarah Holland* – Fertile Mindset

Website: **http://www.fertilemindset.com/eft**

Email: **sarah.fertilemindset@gmail.com**

Tel: +44 (0) 7981 231 392

**Hypnotherapist**

*Lynsi Eastburn* – Hypnofertility

Pioneer in the field of hypnosis for fertility and creator of the HypnoFertility Program

Website: **http://www.hypnofertility.com** or **www.spiritbabywhisperer.com**

Email: **office@hypnodenver.com**

Tel: +1 303 424-2331


## IVF Coordinators (both focused on fertility tourism to the Czech Republic)


### UK – Your IVF Journey

Website: **http://www.yourivfjourney.com**

Email: **info@yourivfjourney.com**

Tel: +44 (0) 115 822 0325


### USA – My IVF Alternative

Website: **http://www.myivfalternative.com**

Email: **info@myivfalternative.com**

Tel: +1 404 324-3955


## Magazines


### My Fertility Specialist (Sheila Lamb)

Fantastic online magazine filled with personal stories, professional information, interviews, tips and all sorts of fantastic fertility related resources.

Website: **http://www.myfertilityspecialist.com**

**Meditations**

*Elisabeth Manning – Baby Spirit Meditation*
Calling in Baby and Nurturing the Spirit
Chakra and Womb Clearing Meditation
Private Baby Spirit Meditation Journey
**http://consciousconception.net/eventsstore**

*Katie Ryan – Fertility Boosting-Mind Body Meditation*
*http://www.katieryan.com.au/free-tools*

*Monica Bivas*
A FREE 3-part guided meditation series for Soulful Women on an IVF Journey
**http://monicabivas.com/en/meditations-series**

*Your Fertile Self*
Customized Meditations Using Your Own Unique Fertility Story. Take a look at **http://www.yourfertileself.com/get-your-fertility-meditation**

Headspace (App Store)
Get Pregnant: Getting Pregnant by Hypnosis (App Store)
Female Fertility: A Self-Hypnosis (App Store)

**Natural Fertility Specialists**

## Andrew Loosely - Natural Fertility Expert

(Lic.OHM, DCHAc.(Beijing), Dip.CH, MURHP, MCMIR)

Andrew Loosely is known as the most sought after Natural Fertility Expert and Consultant in the Fertility community.

He is famous for helping thousands of people around the world to transform their fertility health, and conceive and birth their healthy babies.

Andrew recognises that your delay in conceiving is caused by deeper health factors that need to be addressed before conception can occur naturally or with IVF.

Through his 3-Steps to Pregnancy Programme, The Baby Creating Plan, he supports you to transform your fertility health naturally and increase your chances of natural or IVF conception.

To receive a **FREE** copy of his latest book, **The Ultimate Fertility Guide**, visit: **www.NaturalFertilityExpert.com**
Andrew also hosts the world famous **FREE** online fertility event, **Fertility Question Time.**

You can sign up to over 60 hours of free fertility health support and discussions, by visiting: **www.NaturalFertilityExpert.com/fqt**

## Gabriela Rosa – Natural Fertility Breakthrough

Over the last almost 2 decades Gabriela Rosa MScM (RHHG), BHSc, ND, Post Grad NFM, DBM, Dip Nut, MATMS, MNHAA) and her team have helped bring thousands of healthy babies into the world, even when other treatments have failed.

Gabriela's 7 Step Fertile Method and 11 Pillars of foundations blend the best of both worlds in terms of self-care and science.

This highly experienced team supports couples who have been trying to conceive or experienced recurrent miscarriage for over 2 years—and focuses on natural conception and IVF support treatments to optimise your chances of taking home a healthy baby.

Website: **www.naturalfertilitybreakthrough.com**

Fertility diagnostic quiz to check your fertility score and see what areas you may need to work on for your fertility:

**http://naturalfertilitybreakthrough.com/fertility**

FREE 14 Day Fertility Challenge to begin optimising your chances today:

**http://naturalfertilitybreakthrough.com/fertility-education/14-day-fertility-challenge**

Tel: +61 1300 85 84 90

## *Kate Davies – Your Fertility Journey*

Kate Davies (RN, Bsc (Hons), FP Cert, HS Mgt) is a fertility practitioner, fertility coach and columnist. Kate works with women wishing to optimise their ability to conceive naturally and coaches women going through a difficult fertility journey.

Kate is a registered nurse specialist who, as well as natural fertility, has a special interest in PCOS.

To receive a FREE copy of her book, 50 Tips to Boost Your Fertility visit: **www.yourfertilityjourney.com**

## OTHER

*Bloods 4 You* - **http://www.bloods4you.co.uk**

For ladies/ couples in the UK doing IVF abroad

## *Medichecks* - https://www.medichecks.com

Checks, health screens and blood tests also for ladies in the UK who are doing IVF abroad.

## *FREE IVF Guide for choosing the right Endocrinologist for your IVF treatment*
http://monicabivas.com/en/free-ivf-guide

## *Fertility Jewellery by Monica Bivas*
Gemstone bracelets and necklaces:
http://monicabivas.com/en/fertility-jewelry

# ABOUT THE AUTHOR

Bianca Smith was born in South Africa. She is an IVF veteran, having done 8 IVF transfers between 2013 and 2016. She currently lives in St Pete Beach, Florida where she is loving life with her British-born husband, Vinny, two cats, Fatty & Scruffy and their twin boys, Maximus & Alexei born 20 July 2017 via Surrogacy in Kiev, Ukraine.

**Her subsequent book, My Ukrainian Surrogacy Journey: A Personal Account of My Mission to Motherhood is also available on Amazon.**

She has been writing a (in)fertility blog, **www.wheresmystork.com** since March 2015 with encouraging posts for and by inspirational women, and the following Facebook pages.

Bianca's IVF News & Notes:  facebook.com/**IVFNewsandNotes**

Bianca's Surrogacy News & Notes: facebook.com/**surrogacyinfo**

## HAVE YOU ENJOYED THIS BOOK?

If you have enjoyed this book or found it useful, I would be very grateful if you would post a short review on Amazon.

Your support really does make a difference to an Indy writer like myself.

Thank you again for your support.

Everything I wish I had Known Before Starting My Fertility Treatments

IVF A Detailed Guide available on Amazon in Kindle & Paperback

**& RECENTLY AVAILABLE ON AUDIO (AUDIBLE, AMAZON & iTunes)**

# REFERENCE PAGE

http://www.advancedfertility.com/day3fsh.htm

http://www.advancedfertility.com/hatching.htm

http://www.advancedfertility.com/injections.htm

http://www.advancedfertility.com/ovarstim.htm

http://www.advancedfertility.com/uterus.htm

https://www.arcfertility.com/understanding-embryo-grading/

https://www.asrm.org/BOOKLET_Endometriosis/

https://www.asrm.org/FACTSHEET_Ovarian_Drilling_for_Infertility/

https://www.atlantainfertility.com/Blastocyst-Stage-Embryo

http://www.babycentre.co.uk/a3195/how-to-chart-your-temperature-and-cervical-mucus

http://www.babycentre.co.uk/a549381/ectopic-pregnancy

http://www.bourn-hall-clinic.co.uk/treatments/imsi/

http://www.bourn-hall-clinic.co.uk/treatments/intralipid/

http://www.cmft.nhs.uk/media/1384890/14%2084%20endometrial%20scratch.pdf

http://www.conceivingbyart.com/macs-does-this-procedure-really-help-sperm-quality/

http://www.createhealth.org/fertility-treatments-services/fertility-diagnosis/amh

http://www.createhealth.org/fertility-treatments-services/techniques/embryoscope-time-lapse-imaging

http://www.createhealth.org/fertility-treatments-services/techniques/endometrial-receptivity-array

https://www.dominionfertility.com/fertility-treatment-faq/51-how-can-you-have-an-ectopic-pregnancy-after-ivf/

http://www.drugs.com/pro/solu-medrol.html

http://www.embryoadoption.org/adoption_agencics/embryo_adoption_services_matrix.cfm?CFID=10231980&CFTOKEN=2a1931253e3051ac-783FEE2E-4040-9E6F-F14D03D6B98F559B

http://www.embryoadoption.org/faqs/index.cfm

http://www.embryodonationblog.com/556/do-these-donated-embryos-make-the-grade/

http://www.endometriosisinstitute.com/endometriosis/treatment-of-infertility

https://www.endometriosis-uk.org/your-laparoscopy

https://www.endometriosis-uk.org/sites/default/files/files/Information/laparoscopic_surgery.pdf

https://en.wikipedia.org/wiki/Egg_donation

http://www.fertilityafter40.com/unexplained-infertility.html

http://www.fertilityandgenetics.com/

https://www.fertilityauthority.com/fertility-meds/progesterone

https://www.fertilityauthority.com/fertility-treatment/vitro-fertilization-ivf-explained/assisted-hatching-ivf

http://www.fertilitycenter.com/our_services/infertility_treatments/f
rozen_embryo_transfer/

http://www.ginefiv.co.uk/Magnetic-Activated-Cell-Sorting.aspx

http://haveababy.com/fertility-information/ivf-
authority/interpreting-beta-hcg-pregnancy-test-results

http://haveababy.com/infertility-faqs/beta-hcg

http://haveababy.com/fertility-information/ivf-authority/ivig-
intralipid-therapy-in-ivf-natural-killer-cell-activity-for-diagnosis-and-
treatment

http://www.healthcentre.org.uk/fertility-treatment/picsi.html

http://www.healthline.com/health/semen-analysis#Overview1

http://www.hfea.gov.uk/assisted-hatching.html

http://www.hfea.gov.uk/fertility-treatment-options-reproductive-
immunology.html

http://www.hfea.gov.uk/80.html

http://www.hfea.gov.uk/81.html

http://holisticprimarycare.net/topics/topics-a-g/functional-
medicine/1353-mthfr-mutation-a-missing-piece-in-the-chronic-
disease-puzzle

http://iaac.ca/en/135-556-female-infertility-and-the-thyroid-2

http://www.igenomix.com/tests/endometrial-receptivity-test-era/

http://www.igenomix.com/tests/preimplantation-genetic-
screening-pgs/

http://www.igenomix.com/tests/prevent-genetic-diseases-pgd/

http://www.infertility-guidance.co.uk/blog/2009/03/natural-killer-
cells/

http://www.infertility-guidance.co.uk/fertility_treatments/hysterosalpingography.html

https://www.institutobernabeu.com/en/ib/sperm-retrieval-techniques/

http://www.ivf.com/drilling.html

http://www.ivf1.com/frozen-embryo-transfer/

http://www.ivfconnections.com/forums/content.php/209-Beta-hCG-Values-and-Facts

http://www.ivf-worldwide.com/education/ivf-drug-in-use/ivf-guideline-for-drug-administration/progesterone.html

http://www.ivig.nhs.uk/documents/ivig_patient_guide.pdf

http://www.jillcarnahan.com/2013/05/12/mthfr-gene-mutation-whats-the-big-deal-about-methylation/

http://laivfclinic.com/intravenousimmunoglobulin/

http://www.lifeextension.com/magazine/2009/8/is-homocysteine-making-you-sick/page-01

http://www.rmact.com/getting-started/fertility-testing/day-21-testing

http://www.rmact.com/getting-started/fertility-testing/ovarian-reserve-anti-mullerian-hormone-amh

www.mayoclinic.org/tests-procedures/basal-body-temperature/basics/definition/prc-20019978

http://www.mayoclinic.org/tests-procedures/dilation-and-curettage/basics/definition/prc-20013836

http://www.midlandfertility.com/recurrent-miscarriage-tests/endometrial-scratching/

http://www.midlandfertility.com/recurrent-miscarriage-tests/intralipid-infusion/

http://miscarriage.about.com/od/onetimemiscarriages/p/chemical preg.htm

http://www.mthfrsupport.com.au/what-is-mthfr/

http://natural-fertility-info.com/10-facts-about-sperm.html

http://natural-fertility-info.com/hypothyroidism-reproductive-health.html

http://www.newhealthadvisor.com/LH-Surge-and-Ovulation.html

http://www.nhs.uk/Conditions/Anaemia-iron-deficiency-/Pages/Diagnosis.aspx

http://www.nhs.uk/Conditions/Infertility/Pages/Causes.aspx

http://www.nhs.uk/Conditions/Infertility/Pages/Diagnosis.aspx

http://www.nhs.uk/Conditions/Polycystic-ovarian-syndrome/Pages/Treatment.aspx

http://www.nhs.uk/conditions/pregnancy-and-baby/pages/foods-to-avoid-pregnant.aspx#close

http://www.obgyn.net/endometriosis/association-between-infertility-and-endometriosis-and-treatment

http://www.oxfordfertilityunit.com/treatments-and-pricing/additional-techniques

http://www.pgdlab.com/

http://www.pragueivf.com/en/home/

http://www.preimplantationgeneticdiagnosis.it/

http://www.pregnancycorner.com/loss/chemical-pregnancy.html

http://www.preseed.com/Medical-Professionals/Clinical-Validation/Sperm-Toxicity-of-Nonspermicidal-Lubricant-and-Ultrasound-Gels.aspx

http://www.preseed.co.uk/about-us/

http://www.preventmiscarriage.com/Reproductive-Immunology/Treatment/Humira-Adalimumab-.aspx

http://www.resolve.org/family-building-options/donor-options/embryo-donation-myth-and-facts.html?referrer=https://www.google.co.uk/

http://www.resolve.org/family-building-options/donor-options/using-donor-egg.html?referrer=https://www.google.co.uk/

https://www.rcm.org.uk/news-views-and-analysis/analysis/natural-born-killer

http://www.reproductivemedicineinstitute.com/fertility-treatments/recurrent-pregnancy-loss/pre-implantation

http://www.sart.org/Patients_Guide/

https://www.shadygrovefertility.com/blog/treatments-and-success/ivf-treatment-series-part-one/

http://www.sharedjourney.com/articles/ivig.html

http://www.sims.ie/treatments/testicular-sperm-extraction.1047.html

http://www.theaustralian.com.au/news/immune-system-breakthrough-on-ivf/story-e6frg6n6-1226513987254

http://www.urologyorlando.com/harvesting.html

http://www.vitrolife.com/en/Products/G-SeriesTM-media/EmbryoGlue/

http://www.vitrolife.com/en/Products/EmbryoScope-Time-Lapse-System/

http://www.webmd.com/women/laparoscopic-ovarian-drilling-ovarian-diathermy-for-pcos

http://www.whitelotusclinic.ca/blog/dr-fiona-nd/natural-treatments-for-autoimmune-infertility-concerns/

http://www.womenshealth.ie/pregnancy-clinics-kilkenny-gynaecology-d.asp?ART_ID=9

http://www.yourivfjourney.com/prednisolone-the-fertility-wonder-drug/